SURVIVAL MEDICINE

The Ultimate Prepper's Guide for Medical Emergencies, First Aid, Disasters and Epidemics.

Matthew Coleridge
Copyright © 2020 Matthew Coleridge

All rights reserved.

© Copyright 2020 by Matthew Coleridge
All rights reserved.

This document is geared towards providing exact and reliable information with regard to the topic and issue covered. The publication is sold with the idea that the publisher is not required to render accounting, officially permitted or otherwise qualified services. If advice is necessary, legal or professional, a practiced individual in the profession should be ordered.

From a declaration of principles that were accepted equally by a Committee of the American Bar Association and a Committee of Publishers and Associations.

In no way is it legal to reproduce, duplicate, or transmit any part of this document in either electronic means or printed format. Recording of this publication is strictly prohibited, and any storage of this document is not allowed unless with written permission from the publisher. All rights reserved.

The information provided herein is stated to be truthful and consistent, in that any liability, in terms of inattention or otherwise, by any usage or abuse of any policies, processes, or directions contained within is the solitary and utter responsibility of the recipient reader. Under no circumstances will any legal responsibility or blame be held against the publisher for any reparation, damages, or monetary loss due to the information herein, either directly or indirectly.

Respective authors own all copyrights not held by the publisher.

The information herein is offered for informational purposes solely and is universal as so. The presentation of the information is without a contract or any type of guarantee assurance.

The trademarks that are used are without any consent, and the publication of the trademark is without permission or backing by the trademark owner. All trademarks and brands within this book are for clarifying purposes only and are owned by the owners themselves, not affiliated with this document.

TABLE OF CONTENTS

Chapter 1: First Aid   1

- Life support measures: what is first aid?
- Areas of first aid training
- First aid in traffic accidents
- What is the 4S First Aid Rule?
- First-aid tips
- Your fundamental first resource kit

Chapter 2: Stay calm in emergency situations   11

- Special techniques to train yourself to be calm in catastrophe
- Five steps to better crisis communication
- Be Planned for anything
- Examine the circumstance
- Stay positive
- Much Better Safe Than Sorry- Usage That Code Button!

Chapter 3: First place care of the patient   21

- Really putting patients first: Those with long term conditions
- Key information to put a patient in the first place: Target and guidelines
- Providing information about the funding of GP practices

- The need for honesty and transparency
- Really putting patients first: sharing uncertainty
- Rehabilitation and Intensive Care Strengthening Act: Patients' wishes must come first

Chapter 4: Recognize urgent and emergency situation   30

- Emergency situation – Usage
- Main Difference - Urgent Vs. Emergency
- The urgency care
- The triage comes from emergency situation
- What to do at the time of an emergency?
- How do emergency rooms work?
- Efforts to further improve emergency care
- Managing the Person with Heart Attack in the Emergency scenario
- Extreme urgency: patients with cardiac Emergency: shortness of breath
- The emergency of impotent arterial blood loss
- Kinds of emergencies
1. Primary emergency care
2. Secondary Emergency care
3. Tertiary Emergency care

Chapter 5: First Aid for children   45

- First aid for children: quick action can be crucial
- First measure: address the child and check the breath
- First aid for unconscious children: stable lateral position

- Breathing cessation: Ventilate the child
- Cardiac massage in children
- First aid for children: Treat wounds properly
- Head injuries: Recognize traumatic brain injury
- First aid in case of suffocation
- First aid is a service department for the diagnosis and therapy of medical emergencies
- SHORT-TERM OBSERVATION (OBI)

Chapter 6: Medical support and diagnoses process   52

- Diagnostic Developments
- The healing process for patients
- The Health Care Team

Chapter 7: Infections   59

- Urinary tract infection
- Common liver infections
- Vaginal infection
- Athlete's foot

Chapter 8: Injuries   73

- Small injuries
- Significant injuries
- Soft cells injuries
- Burn injuries
- Head injuries

Chapter 9: Animal bites   88

- Snakebite

- Insects bite as well as stings
- Bee/Wasp Stings
- Fire Ant Bites
- Bedbugs

Chapter 10: Epidemics and viruses — 101

- Pandemic or epidemic
- Influenza epidemics
- Flu
- Ebola
- 1793: Yellow fever from the Caribbean
- 1832-1866: Cholera in three waves
- 1858: Scarlet fever also can be found in waves
- 1906-1907: "Typhoid, Mary."
- 1918: "Spanish influenza."
- 1921-1925: Diphtheria epidemic
- 1916-1955: The height of the polio
- The 1980s to existing: The leading cause of sudden death
- 1981-1991: Measles
- 1993: Polluted water in Milwaukee
- 2010, 2014: Whooping cough
- How to respond to an epidemic situation

Introduction

What is preparedness/survival medication? Our interpretation is: "The practice of medicine in an atmosphere or circumstance where conventional treatment and also centers are not available, typically by persons without official medical training". This consists of medical care while hiking in third world countries, deep-water ocean cruising, separated tramping and also hiking, and also following a huge all-natural catastrophe or various other catastrophes. Everyone should know the essential first aid measures. But be careful: the theory is not the only thing that matters. Only if you regularly train the life-saving handles yourself will they be easy and safe to handle in an emergency! That is why this book recommended. Refresh your first aid knowledge at least every three years with training or a new course.

The basic assumption is that experienced medical professionals, as well as healthcare facility care, will be unavailable for a long term time period, and that along with supplying emergency treatment-- clear-cut treatment as well as recovery (if called for) will require to be offered. Also, the basics of personal as well as public hygiene will certainly additionally require to be considered.

As is the case with any kind of aspects of preparedness, you require to determine what you are getting ready for and also strategy accordingly. For some, it will only be a 72-hour dilemma; for others, it will certainly be a significant lasting occasion, as well as for yet others a numerous generation circumstance. Your medical prep work will certainly need to mirror your own risk evaluations in terms of what understanding and also skills you create and also what supplies/equipment/medicines you store. This publication is much more inclined towards preparation for the tool for longer-term disasters. However, most of them consisted of information that applies to shorter scenarios too.

While the emphasis of this book is on exercising medicine in a survival environment, it does not deal with one essential area which needs to be taken into consideration as part of your prep work. That is optimizing your wellness before any kind of calamity, maintaining fit, keeping a healthy and balanced diet regimen, and also managing any chronic health issue aggressively. This is well covered in 100s of books regarding obtaining fit and also staying healthy and balanced. However, if you do not take some activity in this regard, every one of your other prep work may fail when you drop dead of a cardiac arrest from the anxiety of it all. So this book is the deep within the "Survival Medicine." Allows begin with this publication." An essential book to lead for your first aid in a disaster, epidemics, as well as medical Emergencies."

Chapter 1

FIRST AID

Life support measures: what is first aid?

Those who want to work with children and young people voluntarily, and otherwise, it makes sense to complete it. We are referring to the first aid course.

First aid refers to life-supporting measures that are carried out at an accident site or wherever people are harmed or injured. Unlike the activities of trained rescue workers, first aid measures can be carried out by anyone who is at the scene of an incident with injuries.

Through basic training of private individuals in easy-to-carry out first aid actions, approaching rescue workers can be supported before their arrival, and immediate help can be provided.

What is a first aider?

A first aider is the first person at an accident site who can provide help before the emergency call is made and the emergency services have arrived. This person, therefore, plays a very crucial role in the rescue chain.

Rescue workers often find it difficult or slow to reach an accident site. Even if the scene of the accident can be reached quickly, every minute is precious. Having qualified private first aiders at the scene of the accident is very valuable in this context.

There is sometimes confusion about the exact definition of a first aider. As a rule, every person who first arrives at the scene of the accident is referred to as a first aider. Sometimes, however, only those people who are trained in first aid measures are referred to as first aiders.

First aid training: content & areas

In first aid training, different contents are conveyed, and situations are tested so that a trained person can make the right decisions and take action in an emergency. The areas of the multi-hour course differ depending on the organizer, but usually, always include the same important areas.

Areas of first aid training:

- Immediate measures to save lives: stable lateral position, Heimlich grip, cardiopulmonary resuscitation, handling a mobile defibrillator, etc.

- Drug science: knowledge of typical drugs and some of their side effects and interactions (e.g., ibuprofen, paracetamol, aspirin, nitroglycerin, epinephrine, asthma sprays, etc.)

- Wound care: disinfection, immobilization of parts of the body, handling people when specific injuries are suspected, etc.

- Detection of acute diseases: poisoning, hypoglycemia, heart attacks, strokes, heatstroke, hypothermia, epilepsy, etc.

- Additional knowledge: Knowledge of emergency numbers, ability to secure an accident site, water rescue, psychological support for injured people, etc.

First aid in traffic accidents

In traffic accidents, very large damage can quickly occur, both property damage and personal injury. Traffic accidents also cause traffic jams that make it difficult for rescue workers to reach the scene of the accident. However, since there are usually many people at the scene of the accident, first aid measures can protect the life and limb of those involved in the accident. At the same time, however, there is also a greater risk for local people. Rescuing people from a car is also a particularly big challenge: escaping gasoline can ignite, running engines pose a danger, and injuries can be trapped inside the inaccessible car.

What is the 4S First Aid Rule?

In an emergency, it is not always easy to immediately and correctly remember all the details of the first aid course, which is either long ago or in practice, there was little or no opportunity to implement the learned theory. The 4S rule is a reminder of the four most important steps that must be carried out as part of first aid.

The four S stands for:

- Say you are there and will do something.
- Shielding the emergency victim from onlookers.
- Seek careful physical contact.
- Speak and listen.

First-aid tips

It's necessary to have a well-stocked first useful resource package in your domestic so that you can deal with minor accidents and injuries. Your first useful resource package has to be locked and saved in a cool, dry area out of the attain of children. Many human beings additionally hold a small first resource package in their automobile for emergencies.

Your fundamental first resource kit

A primary first useful resource package might also contain:

- Plasters in a range of exclusive sizes and shapes
- Small, medium and massive sterile gauze dressings
- At least two sterile eye dressings
- Triangular bandages
- Rolled bandages
- Safety pins
- Disposable sterile gloves
- Tweezers
- Scissors

- Alcohol-free cleansing wipes
- Sticky tape
- Thermometer (preferably digital)
- Skin rash creams, such as hydrocortisone or calendula
- Cream or spray to relieve insect bites and stings
- Antiseptic cream
- Painkillers such as paracetamol (or baby paracetamol for children), aspirin (not to be given to youth beneath 16), or ibuprofen
- Cough medicine
- Antihistamine cream or tablets
- Distilled water for cleansing wounds
- Eyewash and eye bath

It may also additionally be beneficial to hold a simple first resource guide or preparation booklet with your first resource kit. Medicines ought to be checked often to make certain they're inside their use-by dates.

Everyone should know that!

Everyone should know the essential first aid measures. But be careful: The theory is not the only thing that matters. Only if you regularly train the life-saving handles yourself will they be easy and safe to handle in an emergency! That is why this book recommended. Refresh your first aid knowledge at least every three years with training or a new course.
And in the meantime, the following tips will help you:

Whatever is right and important! - The package

Whenever you provide first aid, you should follow four very simple steps. With them, you can help everyone injured - and at the same time shorten the time to the arrival of professional help.

Let's summarize these four measures with the term "package"

Constantly check the vital functions of the casualty, call 112 or 110, warm the casualty with a rescue blanket. Also, pay attention to warmth from below. Psychological support: talk to the person concerned, stroke his head. Unconscious people also feel this care.

Not awakenable? - Stable lateral position

An injured man lies ahead of you. He breathes but cannot be awakened, so he is passed out. Now it's time to keep a cool head and do the following:

- The patient must be placed in a stable lateral position. To do this, kneel next to the person affected as a helper. First, take care of the side of the injured person near you. Bend your arm upwards.

- After that comes the far side. Here the arm is placed entirely over the chest, and the distant leg is angled. Now you start at the knee of the bent leg and pull the person concerned towards you. The person concerned then rolls over to your side. Now all you have to do is stretch your head, open your mouth, and put your hands close to the person's body.

In addition to the stable lateral position, it is important to carry out the four measures of the "package": control of the vital functions, emergency call, self-heating, and psychological support.

No breathing? - Cardiac massage and ventilation

The person concerned cannot be awakened and has no more breath. The skin may already have become very pale or blue-grey. A cardiac massage and ventilation must be carried out. The experts speak of "cardiopulmonary resuscitation." To do this, press the center of your chest thirty times, alternating with two breaths - mouth-to-mouth or mouth-to-nose. The "package" must also be observed here - the measures that are always correct. In this case, especially the repeated control of the vital functions and the emergency call.

There are two special features:

In the case of drowning people, it is important to protect themselves first and, therefore, to make the emergency call first. In the event of a power accident, it is important to first disconnect the power supply for your safety. Afterward, if there is no breathing, the heart and lungs should be resuscitated. And: Don't forget the "package"!

Chest problems - Be in the state where your upper body high.

There are many signs by which we can recognize that the injured person has problems in the chest. Shortness of breath, pain, fear, and panic, changes in breathing sounds, sudden coughing attacks, faster and possibly irregular pulse or a pale, sometimes even a blue-grey skin tone suggests this. Symptoms of this type can have many causes.

But in any case, the following applies: The upper body of the injured person must be raised. Tight clothing - ties, shirt buttons, or belts, for example, must be loosened.

In closed rooms, the windows should be opened so that the person concerned gets enough fresh air. Again, the "package" dictates the actions: Check the vital functions, again and again, call for help by phone, maintain the patient's own warmth, and provide care.

The following special features apply in these cases:

If you have an infarction or a cardiac muscle weakness: You can help the person concerned to take preparation previously prescribed by the doctor. It is usually a spray. The same applies to asthma patients. You can often recognize them by rattling noises, especially when exhaling. If an insect stings in the mouth and throat area: It is essential to cool inside and outside! If someone has swallowed something: Then coughing helps. You can help the person affected by tapping lightly between the shoulder blades. It is important to note that the affected person's upper body should be bent down.

Visible injuries - bandage wounds

The main question with injuries is: Are there wounds? They come with three dangers: pain, blood loss, and infection. Important for wounds: wear gloves to protect yourself. Then put on a bandage made of aseptic, suitable material. In the case of heavily bleeding wounds, the injured arm or leg is held up, and the feeding artery is depressed if possible. Does the person have pale, cold skin, dizziness, nausea, and a slow or very fast pulse? He may be in shock. If there are no problems in the chest and no other severe injuries, the patient should be laid flat, and the legs raised slightly.

Foreign bodies in wounds should be carefully removed with tweezers if possible. In the case of more extensive and stuck foreign bodies, the bandage can be put on with padding that reduces the pressure on the foreign body.

The second important question in the case of injuries is: Does the affected person have swelling and pain in the muscles, bones, or joints? Because if this is the case, the corresponding parts of the body must be kept as calm as possible and cooled with an ice pack.
And as always: you should have the "package" with you. So check the vital functions repeatedly, do not forget the emergency call, maintain the injured person's own warmth and - just as important - talk to him and mentally care for him.

Problems in your head - Keep your head up.

Problems in the head can often be clearly seen from external injuries in this area. In addition, sufferers complain of headaches, find it difficult to control their bodies, for example, have memory gaps or paralysis on one side. The most important steps to help are: head up and apply the four actions of the "package" (checking the vital functions, emergency calls, warmth, and psychological care). In the event of a stroke, the paralyzed parts of the body should also be padded. Make sure to provide shade for those affected by sunstroke or heat stroke! In addition, the patient must be cooled - for example, with moist envelopes on the forehead and, if necessary, calf wraps.

Stomach problems? - Knee and neckroll

- In the case of pain in or injuries to the abdomen, it is necessary to provide the person affected with a knee or neck roll to relieve the pain.

- Even if it takes overcoming - sometimes the person affected has to be helped to vomit. In the case of open abdominal injuries, the wound must be treated.

- And, as always, do not forget the "package", the bundle of four actions that are always correct (control of vital functions, emergency calls, warmth, and psychological care).

There are two special features to consider:

If the person affected has diabetes who is insulin-dependent and has hypoglycemia, they also need dextrose! In parallel to the emergency call, you can also contact the Poison Control Center (regionally different number).

Chapter 2

STAY CALM IN EMERGENCY SITUATIONS

Before we talk about what you can do to remain calm and targeted in an emergency, let me inform you why it is vital to continue to be calm and focused. When the physique is underneath stress, it strikes into survival mode, higher acknowledged as the fight-or-flight syndrome. Under these conditions, the physique prepares itself by using overproducing the stress hormone cortisol. Then, cortisol goes to the talent and motives a slow-down in the manner of the pre-frontal cortex, the place you assume significantly, and have your government function. Therefore, the captain of your ship is no longer in control, and the amygdala, the place the combat or flight syndrome, and your feelings come from, receives large and takes over the controls. Finally, the hippocampus, the place your mastering and reminiscence are found, quickly narrows.

So, you can see that, when confronted with an emergency, you are biologically created to be reactive instead of considerate or imperative in your thinking. As a result, panic makes you behave in an emotional manner alternatively than a considerate manner, as you react emotionally to the threat going through you. Because you are no longer residing in primitive society, the place such impulsive and reactive conduct would possibly shop your life. You have to intentionally modify your conduct to accommodate the type of hazard and emergency you are now encountering. And you are at a tremendous downside on every occasion you method any emergency emotionally, instead than logically.

So, you can see that, when confronted with an emergency, you are biologically created to be reactive, as an alternative than considerate or imperative in your thinking. As a result, panic makes you behave in an emotional manner as a substitute than a considerate manner, as you react emotionally to the chance of dealing with you. Because you are no longer dwelling in primitive society, the place such impulsive and reactive conduct may store your life, you have to intentionally modify your conduct to accommodate the type of hazard and emergency you are now encountering. And you are at an awesome drawback each time you strategy any emergency emotionally, instead than logically. As is the case with any kind of aspects of preparedness, you require to determine what you are getting ready for and also strategy accordingly. For some, it will only be a 72-hour dilemma; for others, it will certainly be a significant lasting occasion, as well as for yet others a numerous generation circumstance. Your medical prep work will certainly need to mirror your own risk evaluations in terms of what understanding and also skills you create and also what supplies/equipment/medicines you store. This publication is much more inclined towards preparation for the tool for longer-term disasters. However, most of them consisted of information that applies to shorter scenarios too.

Some rest methods which can assist each you and your young people in case of an emergency include:

Special techniques to train yourself to be calm in disaster

Technique No 1

A rapid modern rest that solely takes a minute of squeezing and releasing all the muscle mass in the physique isometrically and simultaneously, three times, will decrease stress in the physique and right away loosen up you. This technique works best in minor disaster.

Technique No 2

Breathing: Simply taking a minute to breathe into the remember of three, keep to the remember of three, and breathe out to the depend on three, repeated three times, while announcing and focusing every time on the phrase "relax" will robotically calm the mind.

Technique No 3

Create a visualization: Close your eyes for one minute and focal point your idea on some calming cue, for example, a vicinity that you go to relax, a beach, the mountains, and keep that picture three instances to the depend on three. This will minimize your blood pressure, decrease your coronary heart price, and minimize stress. This technique is related to be calm in a disaster situation to low down the high risk of loss.

Technique No 4

An easy Chi Gong physique movement, which can be downloaded for free from any trusted resource online, practiced three times, will center of attention the body, as properly as open up frozen and blocked stress points. This will right away take part off while settling the physique down, as it put you in contact with your bodily self and helps you focus, realizing that your physique is your very own instrument and performs at its fine when built-in with your mind.

When we're overwhelmed

Nobody likes to admit that he or she is overwhelmed with a situation. That is why problems are so often hushed up, hidden, denied - until it no longer works. Desperation and impotence quickly turn into anger at your inability. Only nobody admits this - consequence: The anger is directed outwards. The guilty must be found, while the desperate take refuge in the victim role.

Often it is our own pitfalls that we step into and get excited about things that, when we look closely, are just our interpretation - not necessarily reality. The negative thoughts then become wild speculations and worst-case scenarios, which ultimately culminate in permanent alertness and high blood pressure.

Five steps to deal with any crisis

These steps will help to learn, plan, and implement important ways to deal with disaster or emergency.

Let's have a look in detail:

1. Preparation: Teams, processes, and channels have to be prepared. Who is responsible, who is involved? How are all areas on the go and coordinated at the weekend?

2. Speed along with calmness: Those who are prepared and trained are less likely to lose track even under high pressure. Only with certain calmness can targeted actions and words be defined even during long periods of attendance.

3. Listen and answer: More media, opinion leaders, and platforms lead to an increased burden on the PR position. Comments are waiting for a quick response. Triage becomes difficult - complete silence is impossible. Additional, trained, and informed resources must be used quickly in times of crisis, especially for social platforms.

4. Integrate: All online platforms such as intranet, website, social platforms, and media corner must be compatible with each other. They offer updated information everywhere - in comparison to media conferences, face-to-face meetings, and in the event of longer crises with short-term written means.

5. Plan, improvise and learn: The plan for the disaster was ready, now a new plan is being created every day. It serves as a framework for improvised actions that will always appear. It is important to keep the overall view. You take a lot of coping with each crisis for the next.

Absolutely nothing will truly prepare you for the emotions and truth of an emergency situation dilemma; however, here are numerous tips for maintaining a degree head as well as staying tranquility.

Be Planned for Anything

It's tough to prepare for something that can both never be figured out or provided the level of extent ahead of time. Kinds of emergencies can range from natural calamities, health injuries, and also economic difficulties. Because you will never have the ability to compute when and also just how an emergency situation dilemma will certainly emerge, the most effective suggestions are to be gotten ready for anything and every little thing. Allows state that you were involved in a severe crash, what would occur?

It's a whole lot to think about; however, the last point anybody intends to do throughout an emergency situation crisis is to be agitated over essential yet trivial worries. Instead, you live alone or have a big family member, keeping all this information for emergency situations will certainly aid to relieve several of the mayhem. Produce an emergency situation binder for all family members. Consist of all the important and also the required files that are generally required throughout such occasions. Individual documents, i.e., life insurance policy plans, will & testimonies, as well as also residential property acts. It's constantly far better to be over ready after that adds a considerable boost of panic when whatever is already chaotic.

Examine the Circumstance

Quit, take a breath, and also assume. When emergencies occur, you must have the ability to remove your mind in order to gain access to critical-thinking skills. Panicking will only make the situation worst, so take the last minute to compose on your own and think clearly. When high-stressed scenarios occur, our minds enter a "flight-or-fight" setting. Emotions are enhanced as well as blowing up will just make it worst. Discover a way to promptly soothe yourself as well as focus on what requires occurring following. Ask for emergency assistance, check pulses, stop bleeding, and perform CPR when needed. Once you examine the circumstances of the disaster, this will help to determine the ways to tackle it. Being able to continue to be calm will restrain even more panic and also enable others to comply with lead and also be effective. You keep in mind those fire and twister drills during college? It may have been an exciting break throughout the regular school regimen, yet there was constantly crucial reasoning behind it. We were conditioned to act calm, relaxed as well as adhere to the instructor without worry. Produce a family emergency situation strategy. Does everyone know what to do and also where to go? Having a strategy, as well as a meet up spot, replaces fear with automatic action.

Stay positive

Dwelling on the negatives as well as the thousands of "what-ifs" will just add to the tension of the scenario. Discovering the light and maintaining hope is also the darkest of times will be a welcoming guide. No matter how bad the situation is, bear in mind that it can constantly get worst. Do your best to stay optimistic and favorable by locating coping mechanisms. Ineffective coping is just one of the main reasons that panic arises in high-stress atmospheres. Making a conscious initiative to handle stress levels by staying positive will keep on your own calm and allow you to concentrate on what needs to be done. Imagine all the result situations; acknowledge the most awful, however, make a strategy to aim for the very best. With all the weaves, keep the goal by concentrating on seeing the light.

Be Prepared- Prior to an Emergency situation, Takes place.

See to it you recognize where the code cart/crash cart is when beginning your change. Laying eyes and hands on it prior to you start work is a good way to reinforce its location in your mind, and recognizing where it remains in the instance of an emergency can allow you to react faster, and also provide much better care.

Much Better Safe Than Sorry-- Usage That Code Button!

Experienced registered nurses usually don't call a code till they definitely have to-- they think that they have the skills, experience, and also capacity to care for nearly any kind of client situation. Nonetheless, this isn't always the case, and also keeps in mind-- it's far better to have aid as well as not require it than to need assistance and also not have it. If an emergency situation is establishing, struck that code button. Your client's life depends on it.

Communication and stay calm

Clear communication is crucial in an emergency situation. If you remain in a patient emergency circumstance, you should be talking or paying attention in any way times. Ask other nurses or medical professionals what they require you to do, state what you're doing, ask others if they have executed fundamental jobs (Have you started the IV? Do we need to intubate? By communicating plainly with all workers available while servicing a client, you can mark jobs efficiently and also decrease your very own tension levels. In essence, you will understand exactly what is expected of you, and also have the ability to perform your jobs well.

Why it is really essential to stay calm

Emergency situation conditions can be extremely difficult. An already demanding scenario can be made a whole lot worse when you do not keep your cool. Tension influences the body in countless approaches. With too much stress, the body participates in fight or trip setting by overproducing cortisol-- an anxiety and stress and anxiety hormone. This hormonal agent can create the pre-fontal cortex to decrease, making it difficult to presume plainly, in addition, to feature efficiently. Generally, you have much less control. Do not collapse under pressure; keep your cool with a few of these techniques.

Exactly just how to be calm in an emergency

Maintaining your cool can be hard: Attempt a few of these strategies to cool down, reducing your heart price, and also increase blood flow. Take a step back, in addition, to attempt among these techniques to preserve your calm and be extra convenient than hazardous in an emergency situation.

Take a deep breath: Capture all the muscles in your body concurrently as well as launch as you exhale. Repeat three times. This will certainly increase blood circulation, reduce stress and anxiety, in addition to help to relax you.

Attempt breathing exercises: Take a min to inhale, count to 3, and take a breath out slowly as you count to 3 once more. Repeat three times. Breathing deeply will help to decrease your heart rate, raise blood flow, and also unwind you down.

Close your eyes for a little while, as well as also visualize that you are someplace calming. Photo somewhere guaranteeing like a shoreline, the mountains, or someplace nostalgic to you. Decrease your stress by lowering your heart rate and also decreasing your breathing.

Chapter 3

FIRST PLACE CARE OF THE PATIENT

Local pharmacies are all about health. The experts who advise and sell there are committed to this with knowledge and sensitivity.

Really putting patients first: Those with long-term conditions.

The need for without problems reachable and obvious statistics for sufferers is essential. A current learn about highlights the growing numbers of humans residing with extra than one and frequently numerous lifelong bodily and persistent intellectual conditions. Really placing such sufferer's first means: making sure that such sufferers have continuity of care with a healthcare expert. Whom, the affected person, is aware of and trusts; longer appointments as required; shared selection making and an agreed care plan; and effortless get admission to care. Clinical training, as well as education and learning for non-physicians, can include wilderness medical courses, Lifesaver, and also Armed force Medical Corps training. These courses presuppose that you are providing treatment in the hope of later transporting your client to a functioning clinic, emergency clinic, or field hospital. If you can make the dedication, this training is extremely valuable to have; it's far most likely that you'll experience a short term deficit of medical help than a long term one.

You will certainly likewise need to comprehend just how to deal with specific chronic (serious) medical conditions. Also, a paramedic, for example, is not likely to understand exactly how to deal with an abscessed tooth or a thyroid condition. Most of these problems are treated with medicines and also high modern technology that might no more be readily available.

Let's intend that a tragedy or catastrophe has actually happened, as well as you have actually endured. The power grid is down and is unlikely to be up again for several years. You, however, have prudently saved food, clinical materials, farming, and searching tools, as well as are secure in your sanctuary. You are a penalty, young, strapping person without medical problems and also are sensibly intelligent. Regrettably, you have not the slightest concept of what the first thing is that you must do to ensure your future wellness and also survival. The very first method to help ensure your clinical health is very basic. Do not be a lone wolf! The support of a survival team, even if it's just your extended household, is important if you are to have any type of hope of maintaining it together when points crumble.

There will certainly be tasks that you would discover difficult to think of in an ascetic setting. You will certainly need to stand watch over your residential property. You will certainly need to lug gallons of water from the nearest water resource. You will, eventually, need to chop timber for fuel. Fill a 5-gallon bucket with water and walk 100 yards with it (after staying up from twelve o'clock at night to four a.m. standing outside your house), and also, you'll obtain the feel of what you may need to go with daily.

Being the sole holder of this concern will negatively affect your health and wellness and decrease your opportunities of long-term survival. Worn out and sleep-deprived, you will certainly find yourself a very easy target, not just for looting gangs, yet looting germs. Your body's immune system deteriorates when subjected to lasting stress and anxiety; you will be at threat for illnesses that a well-rested person could quickly weather. However, you cannot. Department of labor and also responsibility will make a difficult situation a lot more workable.

It's not nearly enough to simply remain in a team, nevertheless. Individuals in that team must have normal conferences, decide on concerns, and also set points moving. Put together Strategy A, Plan B, as well as Strategy C and also interact to make their execution effective. Readiness suggests having a plan; have several strategies in place for various turns of occasions. Maintain lines of interaction open to make sure that all your team participants are kept notified.

People with such long-term stipulations and disabilities regularly want to assist and care that crosses regular provider boundaries together with these between important and secondary care, fitness, and social care, as nicely as different carrier areas such as employment, social welfare, and housing. Dealing with specific departments and exclusive companies in specific places is time-ingesting. It can be exceedingly irritating for the affected person who needs to stay as normal a lifestyle as possible. The greater massive availability of the digital affected person report can also help. Though there are nevertheless many difficulties with interoperability, however sharing of the document need to solely be with the categorical permission of the affected person when the facts are being transferred to specific agencies. A pocketbook with current check effects and medicine can be useful with data introduced via each clinician and sufferers who are self-managing. However, possibly, in reality, placing sufferers first ought to imply that the possession of the clinical record, as advised via Sir John Oldham, be transferred from the Secretary of State to the affected person to be stored in protected preserving with the aid of the GP.

Patients trip no longer solely the burden of the ailments; however, additionally, the burden of the treatment. Really placing sufferers first may additionally imply altering offerings so that the affected person can deal without delay with positive services. For example, they are enabling sufferers to hand in specimens without delay to the lab. Due to this fact, the consequences mentioned each to the affected person and the GP. So that the affected person can take motion if required; and making sure that sufferers can have a follow-up go to with an expert. Who considers this critical except the affected person having to go returned to the GP to provoke a new referral, as takes place in some cases.

Key information to put the patient in the first place: Target and guidelines

The NHS and generic exercise are normally revered establishments presenting therapy free at the factor of delivery, however, paid for out of accepted taxation. But sufferers and the public comprehend exceedingly little about how prevalent exercise is organized. The implications of guidelines, protocols, and goals such as QOF (and overall performance management) on how GPs seek advice from work. The fee of the distinctive factors of fitness care and the requirements of care sufferers can expect. Some of these records are in the public area; however, now not constantly comfortably accessible. It is tough to suppose of any different public provider that influences so many of us each day and about which we recognize so little.

Really placing sufferers first requires data for sufferers about the impact of aims such as QOF, protocols, and tips on the work of GPs and their consultations with patients. Quality symptoms such as QOF have a tendency to listen to clinical methods besides enough cognizance of the troubles that are essential to patients —putting sufferer's first need to make certain that indispensable problems in sufferers are blanketed in all nice initiatives. Treatment hints can be mentioned with patients; this is especially essential for sufferers with long-term conditions. Quality additionally consists of the trendy that sufferers can assume from all practitioners. Patients need to be in a position to anticipate that the health practitioner treating them is a properly diagnostician, clinically competent, and up to date. While the introduction of revalidation and Care Quality Commission inspections may additionally provide some indication of quality. The bar for revalidation is low; with restricted significant affected persons enter into the process. Copies of the General Medical Council's Good Medical Practice need to be on view in all practices.

Providing information about the funding of GP practices

Putting sufferer's first ability that sufferers have to recognize how GP practices are funded, including, for example, how lots a GP session costs, the rate of medicines, X-rays, and different investigations, and the repayments for objectives reached. Such statistics ought to be on hand in GP surgical procedures and disseminated via affected person participation companies (PPGs) and NAPP. Some of these records are in the public area; however, now not continually without problems accessible.

Easy availability of such statistics will show that sufferers and the public are being dealt with as accountable adults. The availability of these statistics ought to additionally help affected person and public involvement in commissioning and planning of offerings as nicely as demonstrating accountability.

The need for honesty and transparency

Putting sufferers first potential that gurus and coverage makers are truthful and transparent. Charlotte Williamson discusses how one principal care believes paid GPs to minimize the wide variety of sufferers referred to health center experts and states 'giving economic incentives. The GPs to do something so probably damaging to patients, now not in their pastime and besides prior dialogue, used to be unacceptable'. Many examples of a lack of transparency can be found, such as now not informing sufferers of the black triangle popularity of a medication. This is now not due to wickedness on the section of practitioners, and it is really that the machine has no longer influenced or certainly required the sharing of such records with sufferers and the public. The gadget ought to now change. As the factors out, barring honesty, there can be little admired, and until sufferers are revered, there can be no compassion.

Really putting patients first: sharing uncertainty

I trust that being truthful additionally ability sharing uncertainty with sufferers so that significant (as described by way of the patient) choices can be made. In addition, we, patients, want to respect that the exercise of the medicinal drug is full of uncertainties and that doctors, alternatively equipped and dedicated, are additionally fallible human beings.9 Public and sufferers desire actual possibilities for tremendous involvement in healthcare selection making in the consulting room and at an organizational level. Really placing the sufferer's first need to make this a reality.

A big help - also for families

"It is not a new finding, but health is the most important thing," says the pharmacist, who needs extensive specialist knowledge for his job. He knows the relevant information about active ingredients that are important for the patient. But purchasing, storage, and advertising also require expertise. "The local pharmacy is now important for families because time plays an important role, who is known to many of his small and large customers and can, therefore, select the right products quickly and with the family manager in question for over-the-counter medicines. "We have a lot of regular customers and mostly know their medical history. Over-the-counter medicines are important for health care.

The pharmacist usually recommends them: What is not known to everyone: Doctors can buy over-the-counter medicines on a green.

Prescribe recipe too: With this, the doctor shows that he considers the application necessary from a medical point of view. At the same time, the green serves.

Prescription also as a memory aid: The doctor notes all-important ones on it
Information such as the name of the drug, the pharmaceutical firm, and the pack size.

The patient then redeems it in the pharmacy: By the way: Some statutory health insurance companies reimburse medicines, some of which are prescribed by a green prescription as part of so-called statutory benefits.

Rehabilitation and Intensive Care Strengthening Act: Patients' wishes must come first

On the occasion of tomorrow's hearing on the Rehabilitation and Intensive Care Strengthening Act (RISG), the Joint Association calls for significant improvements. The association criticizes the present draft law as restricting the self-determination and the right to vote of those affected.

"As correct as the introduction of a legal claim to out-of-hospital intensive care is, the planned restrictions on the right to wish and choice of those affected are wrong. If patients are not allowed to choose the place where they are cared for, it would be a blatant violation of the human right to self-determination, "said Prof. Dr. Rolf Rosen rock, Chairman of the Joint Association, with reference to the UN Convention on the Rights of Persons with Disabilities. The choice is for the well-groomed, their relatives, or legal care.

The introduction of a new independent entitlement to intensive care outside the clinic and the anchoring of the "rehabilitation before care" principle in rehabilitation services is to be welcomed in principle. However, the joint venture also sees a need for improvement in the details of other regulations, including invasive ventilation and weaning in hospitals. According to the association, there is a lack of equipment and structures across the board. "Unfortunately, there is still a lack of specialist staff and weaning centers across the board.

Chapter 4

RECOGNIZE URGENT AND EMERGENCY SITUATION

Emergency situation refers to significant and also oftentimes the dangerous happenings need immediate focus. Urgent is an adjective that defines some issues trying out the place motion or interest. As a result, these expressions have the very same definition. However, their use in sentences is lovely as a result of the truth; they come from 2 remarkable grammatical categories.

Covered primary areas

- What is urgency mean?
- What does emergency mean to you?
- What are all the stylistic similarities among both urgent and also emergency situations?
- What is the distinction between Urgent and Emergency situations?

Emergency situation – Usage

The phrase emergency is a noun that describes an unanticipated, on a regular basis, and an unpredictable scenario requiring instant activity. For instance, a mishap, which takes location suddenly, as well as which needs fast action to handle it. Additional care is an abrupt health circumstance like a stroke or stroke. Along with these, all-natural calamities like quakes, floods, wildfires, hurricanes, tidal waves, and so on are furthermore emergency situation scenarios.

Main Difference - Urgent Vs. Emergency

Generally, an emergency presents a right away hazard to life, health, and wellness, building, or setting. We usually identify the cops, health department, fire brigade, or another well-trained volunteer in case of an emergency. Similarly, an emergency ward is a ward in a mental hospital that absorbs sufferers who need instantly care.

The urgency care

The term triage originates from the French word "trier," as well as indicates "type." It describes the process of assessing the urgency of treatment for emergency patients. Specialists must recognize the importance of immediate treatment based on vital signs such as blood pressure and temperature, as well as statements and symptoms from the patient within a few minutes.

The triage comes from emergency situation

The triage originally comes from emergency situation, which regulates a mass casualty situation. Helpers divide the injured into different groups:

- Red: an acute threat to life: immediate treatment
- Yellow: seriously injured: postponed treatment

- Green: slightly injured: later treatment
- Blue: no chance of survival: wait-and-see treatment

The disaster management system is not transferable one-to-one to the emergency room. Otherwise, dying patients would receive a blue sticker, and the doctors would no longer treat them. In contrast, no patient may be rejected in the emergency room.

What to do at the time of an emergency?

In the treatment landscape (emergency), there are various assistance and treatment offers for individuals with some urgent health issues. Which makes sense relies on the kind and intensity of the symptoms. It is not easy for a layperson to distinguish in some situations, whether it is a real emergency or not. An emergency is generally assumed if there is a risk to life or permanent damage cannot be excluded. These include, for example, serious accidents, suspected stroke or heart attack, severe blood loss, and similar situations. Then it is clear: Dial 112 immediately or go to a rescue center.
Otherwise, if possible, first contact your family doctor. If you are unsure, at night, at the weekend or on public holidays, when there is no practice open, and the doctor's visit cannot be postponed, the medical on-call service of the statutory health insurance associations (also called emergency or emergency service) helps. He can be reached on the free number 116117. Callers are automatically redirected to the central office responsible for their place of residence. The medical staff of the emergency service assesses whether someone urgently needs help, a home visit is necessary or whether the

patient should go to so-called emergency practice. If the doctor's visit cannot wait until the next working day, general practitioners and specialists treat you outside of regular office hours in over 600 on-call offices across Germany. The medical on-call service looks after health insurance and private patients.

How do emergency rooms work?

In an emergency room, specialist's generally first check which cases are urgent and need to be treated immediately using vital signs such as breathing, pulse, blood pressure, body temperature, and the symptoms and information provided by the patient. Some hospitals classify the patients into different color groups: red for life-threatening patients, yellow for seriously injured, and green for slightly injured. Others work with a five-stage system with the colors red, orange, yellow, green, and blue, red being immediate treatment and blue being non-urgent. It is, therefore, important to provide clear information about the health complaints directly when registering.

A doctor examines the patient and decides on treatment. Depending on the diagnosis, the patient is referred to as the responsible specialist department or can be dismissed home with a doctor's recommendation.

Efforts to further improve emergency care

For years, more and more patients with mundane everyday complaints have been going to the overloaded rescue centers, which are affiliated to the hospitals and are intended for medical emergencies. This costs hospitals a lot of money; the non-emergencies block the lines of the emergency service 112 and hinder or delay the timely handling of urgent emergencies.

New regulation of emergency care should remedy this. It is planned to organize outpatient and inpatient emergency care centrally "under one roof." Joint emergency control centers are used to direct patients to the right place, i.e., to either refer them to a hospital or the family doctor on call. In addition, inpatient emergency care is to be restructured. Hospitals will, in the future, be graded according to emergency levels and must meet certain minimum requirements.

Managing the Person with Heart Attack in the Emergency scenario

Heart attack (HF) is an around the world public health concern influencing approximately 26 million individuals worldwide. It is the leading source of a medical facility stay in the U.S.A. as well as Europe. Individuals hospitalized with HF have a higher in-hospital and post-discharge death in addition to an enhanced rate of re-hospitalizations. As numerous as 77% of these individuals at the first discussion to the emergency department (ED), posturing countless challenges. These include the requirement for fast clinical diagnosis incorporated with a very early shipment of appropriate treatment along with danger stratification to help the appropriate individual character.

Cardiac arrest individuals may offer to the ED with differing expert situations, each connected with particular clinical functions. Serious HF, defined as the fast beginning of signs as well as signs second to uncommon heart feature, may supply as extreme lung oedema in addition to hypertension (vasoactive), shock, absence of breath, or oedema with liquid overload. Heart disorder can be connected with the systolic or diastolic disorder, valvular disorder, or separated ideal ventricular disorder. While serious HF can offer without previously recognized heart dysfunction, 63% 7 to 75% 5 has a diagnosis of HF before the discussion.

It is necessary to acknowledge, along with managing speeding up elements early. The 2016 European Society of Cardiology (ESC) HF Requirements highlights coronary condition, high blood pressure, arrhythmia, mechanical problems, as well as pulmonary emboli (phrase CHAMP) as medical diagnoses that need to be dismissed early in the evaluation. While coronary artery disease is common among clients with decompensated HF, evaluating for anemia in people with new-onset HF is underutilized. Various other reasons for decompensating such as blood loss, infection, as well as additionally thyroid disorder also need to be determined immediately as well as treated.

The therapy of HF in the ED entails synchronized 'usual' HF therapy and also element to consider of the speeding up variables. After first stabilizing, present standards suggest treatment with diuretics, vasodilators, or inotropes based upon clinical hemodynamic accounts. The evidence base for extreme HF therapy is restricted as well as presently, the only Course I suggest for clinical treatment in intense HF is intravenous technicality diuretics in clients with fluid overload (LOE C). In individuals without hypotension, intravenous vasodilators (such as nitroglycerine) should be considered and also perhaps the first line in those with high blood pressure.

An essential aspect of the therapy in the ED, after the medical diagnosis, as well as the initiation of treatment, is the choice of correct personality. This should certainly be based upon the specific person's danger stratification. To assist this analysis, the ED doctor can connect with the cardiologist, ideally an HF expert. Included valuable information might be gathered by straight contact with the health care physician or referring cardiologist.

A hospital stay in HF can be utilized for analysis workup, improving signs as well as likewise volume overload, treatment of precipitating components along with existing together diagnoses, releasing standard directed treatment for chronic HF, and also customizing recurring medical management as well as a social aid.

Extreme urgency: patients with cardiac

Cardiac arrest (HF) is a worldwide public health issue influencing approximately 26 million individuals worldwide. It is the leading root cause of a hospital stay in the USA as well as Europe. Certainly, patients with cardiac or needing ventilator assistance, 83.7% of American clients from the Nationwide Emergency Department Example (NEDS) information source with a main ED medical diagnosis of extreme HF were hospitalized. With the disease, medically called heart failure, the heart muscle can no longer pump the required amount of blood through the heart to supply the organs. The reduced pump function can be caused both by a problem with contraction of the heart muscle (systolic heart failure) and by the fact that the left ventricle is not sufficiently filled with blood (diastolic heart failure). Heart failure can be caused by, among other things, coronary heart disease (CHD). Complaints can include shortness of breath when climbing stairs, water retention, cardiac arrhythmias, or difficulty breathing even when at rest.

In order to better care for patients with heart failure, the Clinic for Cardiology, Angiology, and Pneumology at the Heidelberg University Hospital called under the project management of Professor Dr. Lutz Frankenstein launched the project "HeiTel: Telemedical care for patients with heart failure" in 2006 together with the AOK Baden-Württemberg. The project was preceded by the randomized study "HITEL," in which 100 patients were examined in three groups over a period of one year. The first study group received standard care from the family doctor; the second group received standard care, including telemedical care, and the third group received care from the university clinic with telemedical care. "In the project, we were able to show that the hospitalizations and the drug compliance of the third group have improved significantly. And also, the titration of the medication, which is very relevant for heart failure, could be dosed in the target range recommended in the guidelines", explains Professor Frankenstein. According to Frankenstein, it is a known problem that patients receive the right medication, such as beta-blockers or ACE inhibitors, but they are not administered in the correct dose. Studies on this, however, show that patients with an exact titration live longer.

Finally, HF is a substantial origin of a medical facility stay, and additionally, great deals of the patients are confessed by means of the ED. It could give various medical situations. Medical diagnosis is testing, as well as the need to be developed promptly using many easily available gadgets. An examination seeking precipitating components requires to be done all at once. Treatment includes extremely early maintenance based upon hemodynamic accounts, along with taking care of the accelerating component if one can be determined. Customer triage, in addition to character, is based upon the approximated danger, utilizing a tracking system if required, and also assuring continuous treatment in the outpatient setting.

Emergency: shortness of breath

In medical terms, shortness of breath is referred to as dyspnea. There are many possible causes: In addition to obstruction of the airways by foreign bodies, various diseases can be behind it. In general, a distinction is made between shortness of breath that only occurs during physical activity and shortness of breath that is also noticeable in rest situations. The severity of breathlessness depends on many factors and is perceived differently subjectively. In any case, it is important to recognize the signs and act accordingly. Severe shortness of breath is always an emergency. In this situation, you must act quickly as a first aider and immediately call 911 if you experience the following symptoms:

- Rapid breathing
- Pale and bluish-gray skin, especially in the lips, nails or eyelids

- Breathing noises such as whistling, rattling, wheezing
- Increased breathing and support of the upper body (e.g., stopping at the back of a chair or the edge of a table) in order to use the auxiliary breathing muscles
- Sudden cough
- Inability to speak as well
- Cold sweat, fear of death

In the event of severe shortness of breath, it is important to dial emergency number 144 immediately. The focus is then on reducing stress. All supporting measures, e.g., soothing conversations, help in this emergency situation. Calm the person down, and try to stay calm yourself. The person concerned should sit or be placed with a raised upper body. Bracing your arms makes breathing easier. Under no circumstances should she/he move. Open tight clothing and provide fresh air. Monitor the condition of the person concerned.

In the event of loss of consciousness or sudden loss of consciousness: Call out for help and make people in the area aware of the emergency situation! Check awareness (speak and gently touch). Check to breathe: hear, see, and feel for max. Ten seconds: As long as there is still breathing: Bring the victim to the stable side position and dial the emergency call. Check to breathe again! If there is no normal breathing, then call 144 immediately. The main causes of shortness of breath are either in airways (throat, trachea, and bronchial tubes), the heart, or the lungs. Other reasons can be muscle disease, anemia, injuries, or tumors.

When faced with a person in respiratory system distress or uneasiness, the immediate care of the patient is essential. Initially, one needs to establish if the individual remains in the respiratory system worry, in spite of the underlying cause. Cyanosis, agonal breathing, overstated breast wall surface activity without simultaneous air activity with mouth or nares might quickly suggestions to developing this. If apprehension impends, then we abide by the recoup mouth to mouth resuscitation standards of compressions, safeguarding a respiratory system and additional airflow, due to order. Or else if hand-operated breast compressions are not called for in the individual, after that, we should attempt to recognize the start of the respiratory system distress.

Problem breathing from breathing system clog can take place from the exterior nares, nasal flows, throat, bronchi, and also down to little bronchioles. Many factors can activate the respiratory tract to become obstructed: foreign body, vomit or hemorrhage, neoplastic, swelling or edema, injury from cracks of the skull or throat, hematoma formation, along with brachycephalic conformation.

Difficulty breathing can similarly take place due to the failure of the lungs to raise, developing the lung to collapse. This makes it difficult for the lungs to relocate air right into the alveoli as well as to enable the gas exchange to take place. Damages to the CNS can affect the breathing system facilities in the mind and also effective control of the diaphragm.

When the lung cannot obtain oxygen from the lot more significant respiratory systems after that, gas exchange is undoubtedly damaged. It becomes a cause and effect. In essence, the lung can't acquire oxygen; gas exchange cannot happen in between the lung right into the blood; the body detects it is not getting adequate oxygen. So it increases the respiratory system as well as initiative effort to maintain the crucial body organs oxygenated. This enhanced initiative is why we see noticeable breast wall surface area motion in heart trouble with lung edema and pneumonia. There are some circumstances where lung function is normal, yet blood circulation to the lungs is impaired, as well as additionally, oxygen can't get in the circulation. Injury to the vessels in the lungs, as well as embolism (lung thromboembolism), is two typical factors for this emergency breathe arrest.

The emergency of impotent arterial blood loss

A wound that is deep, hemorrhaging considerably, or has blood streaming from it (activated by hemorrhaging from an artery), may not clot and likewise may not give up blood loss.

1. Call out for a person to obtain help or call 911 by yourself. Do not get rid of a pad that is soaked through with blood; you will definitely interrupt any type of kind of embolism that has actually started to create to aid give up the blood loss. If blood soaks through, area an additional pads in addition to the saturated one, in addition, to continue applying direct anxiety.

2. When the blood loss decreases or stops. Then use the pad, tie tight with gauze strips, or a lace. Do not connect so snugly that blood circulation to the remainder of the arm or leg is removed. Stay with

the individual as well as keep the injury elevated until the ambulance gets in.

If significant bleeding does not stop with straight anxiety as well as also altitude, apply straight pressure to an artery—straight usage stress on an artery together with altitude and straight tension on the injury. There are specific considerable arteries in the body where tension needs to be put. If there is serious blood loss, additionally use firm pressure directly to the hemorrhage. In the event of heart as well as likewise respiratory system apprehension, begin promptly with prompt procedures (airflow as well as heart massage therapy). Begin airflow to guarantee that the oxygen supply in the blood is shielded.

Kinds of emergencies

Primary emergency care

Lots of people face with the primary emergency. This is your initial as well as also most generalized stop for signs and symptoms as well as professional troubles. For instance, you might see your health care doctor when you observe any sign or worried that you got the flu, or some other microbial or viral ailment. You may, in addition, choose healthcare for a broken bone, a hurting muscle mass, a skin rash, bleeding, shattered arm or legs, serious burned, poisoning, or any other intense clinical concern. In addition, health care is typically in charge of collaborating your care among professionals, in addition to other medical care.

Treatment carriers (PCP) might be physicians, nurse practitioners, or professional medical assistants. There is some healthcare specialized too. Study studies have actually revealed that healthcare firms benefit the healthcare system simultaneously by offering boosted accessibility to medical care services, far better health and wellness results, and a decrease in a hospital stay and also use emergency department visits.

Secondary Emergency care

When your primary emergency care refers you to an expert, you are after that in secondary emergency care. Secondary emergency care specialists primarily concentrate either on a particular system of the body or a particular condition or problem. Like for instance, cardiologists treat any heart as well as its pumping system. Endocrinologists concentrate on hormonal agent systems, and some focus on illnesses like diabetes mellitus or thyroid disease. Oncologists have specialized in treating cancers cells, and also numerous focuses on a particular sort of cancer cells.

Additional emergency situation care is where many people wind up when they have a medical condition to handle that cannot go to the primary emergency treatment level. Your doctor might call for that you obtain a recommendation from your PCP before going directly to a professional. A second emergency situation includes a few of the adhering to emergencies, e.g., head trauma, subjected damaged limbs and presumed damaged hip bone, and so on. There are times when issues with specialty treatment establish. You may likewise experience problems having more than one professional if each is taking care of various troubles. In these situations, your treatment may not be coordinated.

Tertiary Emergency care

As soon as a patient is hospitalized, he needs a greater degree of specialty care in an emergency situation within the medical facility; he may be referred to as tertiary emergency situation treatment. Tertiary emergency situation care calls for highly specialized equipment and know-how. At this level, you will absolutely find treatments such as coronary artery bypass surgical treatment, kidney, or hemodialysis, along with some cosmetic surgeries or neurosurgeries.

It likewise includes extreme shed treatments, no significant injuries, little burned, damaged limbs not subjected, as well as any other very intricate treatments or procedures. Studies have actually revealed that in the management of some persistent issues such as diabetic issues and persistent kidney disease, it is still crucial for the primary emergency treatment service provider to be included when a client goes into tertiary emergency treatment. Having the PCP included might improve lasting self-management by the individual.

Chapter 5

FIRST AID FOR CHILDREN

Rapid action is required in the event of an accident. First aid for children has a few special features. Since parents are often the first to be on-site, they should know what to look out for when providing primary care for children after an accident.

First aid for children: quick action can be crucial

The majority of all child accidents happen at home. Therefore, it is usually the parents who are given the role of first aiders. However, many mothers and fathers are afraid of injuring the child and therefore prefer not to do anything. A sometimes dangerous mistake - because it often takes too long for an ambulance to arrive. During this time, serious damage can occur, which can be avoided by first aid to the child.

An example: The brain only needs about three to five minutes without oxygen. Ventilation can, therefore, be elementary to bridge the time until professional help is on site. There are special courses for parents that teach first aid to children. They are recommended for all parents to learn the measures in practice and to lose the fear of mistakes.

First measure: address the child and check the breath

If your child is lying motionless on the floor, you should first speak to and touch them. Check if it responds. But don't pull it up - you could hurt it even more. At best, the child can explain what happened to you. Then you can treat it accordingly, for example, with a bandage.

If the child does not respond, you or another person present should dial 112. Until support arrives, you should take action yourself and provide the child with first aid. Check his breath first. To do this, gently bend the child's head back slightly and open his mouth. Try to hear and feel the breath. Caution: If you need to provide first aid to a baby, be careful not to stretch your head.

First aid for unconscious children: stable lateral position

If the child breathes, that's a good sign. You should then immediately bring it to the stable side position. If it is on its back, it could vomit and suffocate. For a stable side position, turn the child on its side. The lower leg is stretched out long; the upper leg is bent. The lower arm is angled with the palm facing up; the upper arm is crossed over it. The child's head is tilted slightly backward. Make sure that your mouth is open so that vomit or blood can drain and not get into the airways.
In a baby, the stable side position looks a little different: lay the baby on its stomach, turn its head to the side and open its mouth.

If the child is lying stable, cover it up and watch it until a doctor or medic arrives. If the child regains consciousness in the meantime, it should, if possible, remain in this position until the emergency services are on site. Speak calmly and clearly with him, tell him that help is coming soon and stroke the child - so it feels that it is not alone and rather stays calm.

Breathing cessation: Ventilate the child

If you cannot find breathing, you must give the child breath. To do this, breathe in normally and hold the child's nose shut. Then blow air into the child's mouth until the chest rises. Release your nose again. Keep in mind that children's lungs are smaller and can hold less air. When the chest sinks again, breath again. Repeat at least five times.
There is a peculiarity when breathing a baby: Here, you have to ventilate your mouth and nose at the same time. As soon as the child begins to breathe again, you can put it on its side.

Cardiac massage in children

If ventilation is unsuccessful, you should start cardiac massage immediately. If you are supposed to treat a child over the age of one. Just place your palm on the lower area of the breastbone. Push the breastbone down two to four centimeters (depending on the size of the child) 30 times. Try to keep a frequency per minute compression about 100 to 120. Then perform two ventilations. You always continue this procedure alternately. As soon as the child breathes himself, bring him to the stable side position. When giving first aid to a baby, use only two fingers for the cardiac massage, not the entire ball of the hand.

First aid for children: Treat wounds properly

A small bicycle accident cut your finger while cooking or got stuck on an obstacle while romping: It is not uncommon for children to bleed as a result of injuries. The shock is great at first, but you should stay calm. Take a close look at the wound and see how serious it is. The first impression can be mislead by blood smeared over a large area. Deep or extensive injuries often need to be sewn. In such a case, you should see a doctor or a hospital.

You can treat smaller wounds yourself. Pay particular attention to cleanliness, and wear disposable gloves. First, clean the wound with water. If the injury is bleeding easily, a patch is sufficient. You can stop heavy bleeding with a pressure bandage: To do this, place a sterile compress on the skin of the small patient and a pressure pad over it. You fix this with a gauze bandage.

Head injuries: Recognize traumatic brain injury

In the event of a fall, children often hit their heads hard. Often it remains a small bump. Then a cooling compress helps against the swelling. Sometimes there is a laceration or even a traumatic brain injury. Pay attention to whether the child is extremely tired or is vomiting after a head impact. Both can indicate a concussion. Even if a child passes out after a fall, traumatic brain injury is likely. Bring him to the side and call 112. If the child is not breathing, apply ventilation and, if necessary, cardiac massage.

First aid in case of suffocation

Small children are only too happy to put objects in their mouths. If they get into the trachea, it becomes dangerous. Usually there is a cough and gagging, which in the best case ensures that the foreign body is transported out again. However, if the child has difficulty breathing or produces whistling noises, you should act quickly. In severe cases, the child turns blue or even passes out.
Immediately ask the child to cough vigorously. If that doesn't reveal the swallowed item, try loosening it up to five times between the shoulder blades. Bend the child's upper body forward. In an emergency, call the ambulance service and use the so-called Heimlich handle: embrace the child with both arms from behind and place your hands between the navel and sternum. Pull jerkily a few times so that pressure is exerted on the upper abdomen. However, the handle can cause injuries and should, therefore, only be used in emergencies.

First aid is a service department for the diagnosis and therapy of medical emergencies

The children are accompanied by the general first aid in the pediatric first aid, which is accessible 24/24 hours without a reservation. It is very important to us that the patients receive the best possible care in the shortest possible time, depending on their condition and requirements. The little patients are still being examined for urgency.
The first aid service should only be consulted in urgent cases. Excessive crowds in pediatric first aid prevent nurses and doctors from correctly evaluating, treating, and caring for young patients. For problems that are not

really urgent, the pediatrician should be consulted during the day, while the emergency medical service is available at night and on public holidays.

SHORT-TERM OBSERVATION (OBI):

Possibility of observation for acute symptoms that require longer nursing and therapeutic measures. This service can be used for 36 hours.

No life-threatening situation

Call the pediatrician or the national emergency number of the National Association of Statutory Health Insurance Physicians on the nationwide telephone number 116 117. Here parents can ask for advice if they are unsure whether to go to the emergency room of a clinic. They also find out where the next open standby practice is. In large cities, in particular, parents have to expect long waiting times in an emergency room - if their concern is not serious. Because: "Patients are urged for urgency."

Life-threatening situation

Dial 112 for the ambulance and emergency doctor. Anyone who doubts whether this is really necessary should do so. Because the rescue control center decides whether to send a car. There are no costs for this. Even if the emergency doctor comes for free, because the child is now better off, parents do not have to pay for the operation. "If a child is passed out and needs to be resuscitated, the control center gives precise instructions on how to do cardiac massage and ventilation," says Florian Hoffmann. A big request to all parents and guardians: brush up on your knowledge of first aid in a special course for babies and children.

Chapter 6

MEDICAL SUPPORT AND DIAGNOSES PROCESS

College of Southampton spinout High field Diagnostics will certainly advertise a brand-new modern technology at the 2019 Consumer Electronic Devices Show that is readied to change the concept of 'instantaneous' medical diagnostics.

Scientists from the College's Optoelectronics Study Centre have actually created the world's first non-reusable test. That can simultaneously perform separate medical diagnoses, allowing the screening of diseases or problems such as tuberculosis, sexually transferred infections, or leishmania, a parasitic disease comparable to jungle fever, from a single sample.

"This basic and rapid screening stands for genuine innovation in global healthcare surveillance as well as a medical diagnosis in residence, the physician's surgical procedure or even off-grid rural settings in developing nations," founder Teacher Robert Eason describes. "The fast diagnostics market is truly global. If we simply took into consideration the instance of tuberculosis, there are 10 million people who are presently presenting energetic signs and symptoms in India as well as more two billion individuals worldwide who currently harbor the condition in its hidden form."

High field Diagnostics can produce tests that reveal an increase of the level of sensitivity of an element of one hundred contrasted to existing standard examinations, so individuals can recognize much earlier if they are struggling with a certain problem.

The team is likewise capable of creating tests that provide measurable results such as the low, medium, or high visibility of a defined disease, which represents an action change to present pregnancy examinations, for instance, that are just able to give a yes or no result.

Diagnostic Developments

The array and capacity of analysis tests are constantly progressing, aiding to identify diseases earlier, in more information, and also across more regions of the globe. In this checklist, we have a look at seven appealing developments in the analysis of modern technologies from 2017.

A Mass Spec Pen to Quickly Determine Cancer

One of the biggest obstacles of cancer surgical procedure is making certain that all traces of the cancer are eliminated while preserving as much healthy and balanced cells as feasible. The success of this could be significantly improved with a brand-new device just recently established by scientists at The University of Texas at Austin.

In simply 10 seconds, the Mass Spec Pen can properly recognize cancerous cells throughout surgery, with over

96% precision. The pen functions by evaluating metabolites from the cells, which vary between regular as well as cancerous cells. It is really hoped the technology will begin evaluating in surgical treatment in 2018.

Paper Point-of-Care Zika Test

Populace screening can play a vital duty in detecting and also taking care of Zika, identifying the presence of the condition prior to signs appears. This relies upon access to inexpensive and straightforward examinations, which can be made use of in resource-limited settings.

Researchers from Washington University in St. Louis are developing such a test. Made from paper, the examination setting you back roughly 10 to 15 cents, creates a color adjustment when immunoglobins in the blood of an infected patient respond with small gold Nanorods on the paper. A unique Nanocrystal layer supplies defense to the test throughout the delivery as well as storage.

Transparent Cells for Pathological Diagnosis

Conventional methods of pathological diagnosis rely upon staining slim areas of person specimens. Imaging in 3D might get over some of the restrictions related to this technique, as well as help pathologists discover abnormalities that may otherwise have actually been missed out on.

A current study has actually demonstrated that CUBIC (Clear, Unblocked Brain/Body Imaging Cocktails, and Computational Analysis) works at defining normal and also unusual regions in lung and also lymph node tissues. The appealing results highlight the potential for 3D histopathology to enhance medical diagnosis treatments.

Self-powered, Paper-based Electrochemical Diagnostics

Point-of-care diagnostics, which are mobile, inexpensive, as well as call for the little framework, can help to enhance health care in areas with limited access to extra innovative research laboratory devices.

SPEDs (Self-powered, Paper-based Electrochemical Devices), just recently created at Purdue University, offer a variety of advantages for individuals in remote regions or military bases. Made from paper, the cost-effective devices are lightweight and also versatile, as well as can test for a variety of illnesses without requiring an expert user.

A Microfluidic Chip to Anticipate Preterm Birth

Identifying expectant females in jeopardy of preterm birth might allow earlier interventions to help postpone birth and enhance the infant's lungs, minimizing the chances of morbidity as well as death.

A freshly created integrated chip can focus, separate, as well as spot little quantities of P1 peptide in a blood example. P1 can suggest an enhanced threat of preterm birth, so the chip can eventually be used in healthcare setups to determine expecting females that may take advantage of clinical interventions.

Smartphone TRI Analyzer

A rising number of diagnostic tools are being established for usage with smartphones, a result of their widespread presence, ease-of-use, and also expanding power and also capabilities.

Established by researchers at the College of Illinois at Urbana-Champaign, the TRI (Transmission, Reflection as well as Intensity Spectral) analyzer is the initial portable device able to do three of one of the most common types of examinations in clinical diagnostics, utilizing a smartphone's inner rear-facing camera as a spectrometer.

A Wearable Sweat Sensor

Sweat is an appealing biofluid for non-invasive diagnostics, having a number of solutes that can serve as biomarkers for health and disease.

After promoting the skin to produce tiny amounts of sweat, a brand-new wearable sweat sensor finds the molecules and also ions existing, and afterward sends out the data to a web server for analysis. The sensor has been made use of in researches to find chloride ions, which might lead to enhancements in detecting cystic fibrosis.

The healing process for patients

Every patient has a one-of-a-kind see and therapy program specific to his/her condition. Nevertheless, similar to you have an everyday routine in your home, there is additionally a foreseeable rhythm to medical facility activities. Even though a healthcare facility is a place of rest and recovery, it's a really busy place. Recognizing what to anticipate will help you choose the most effective possible time for your browse through.

Provided here are some regular activities that create the normal ups and downs of medical facility activity from the patient's viewpoint:

The Health Care Team

Along with the routine day-to-day activities, a patient receives treatment from a number of various carriers in their healthcare group. The local time these team members connect with an individual may vary, relying on schedules. Occasionally working with every person's needs as well as agendas can be made complex.

Remote Assistance

There are 2 points you can do even if you can't make it to the healthcare facility or live out of the community. Discover exactly how you can take advantage of the cost-free services available for you to connect with your loved one. Or you can buy presents and blossoms from our present shop.

Examining vital signs: Many tasks are arranged during the day so a patient can rest at night. Checking essential indications (high blood pressure, temperature, pulse, and also breathing rate) is an exemption. From admission to discharge, many clients have their important signs inspected on a daily basis continuously.

Lab technicians: Lab technicians will take blood examples very early. The team uses the essential signs as well as laboratory results from the blood sample to make or readjust their preparation for a patient.

Meals: Nourishment is a popular time for patients as well as their friends and family. You can get a visitor meal as well as consume with your relative or close friend. Mealtimes are staggered; however, typically take place around the expected times-- early morning, afternoon, and also night. Contact your patient's device nurse to get a more precise time of when your close friend or family member will certainly be offered.

Personal treatment: At some time throughout the first half of the day, individual care help will certainly be provided for those who require it. This consists of assistance with activities such as cleaning teeth as well as hair, face cleaning, showering, and also making use of the bathroom.

Drugs: Registered nurses carry out drugs to each patient based upon the timetable suggested by the medical professional. This timetable doesn't always correspond to any other activities.

House cleaning: House cleaning will enter into a patient's space once or twice a day to empty rubbish, clean the shower rooms, wipe down sinks as well as usually maintain every little thing gleaming and organized. They have to adhere to lots of regulations to make certain whatever is cleaned up according to strict requirements.

Chapter 7

INFECTIONS

Infections that generally come as a result of bad cleanliness as well as health, such as diarrheal condition and body lice. There are many various other types of bacterial, viral, as well as the parasitic condition that might not necessarily have sanitation and hygiene as a factor, but can be as dangerous. Appendicitis, as an example, can happen in anybody despite their tidiness or the problems at their retreat. A basic in-grown hair may result in a boil or abscess.

Our bodies' all-natural capacity to eliminate illness goes over. There are, nonetheless, nobody organs that are unsusceptible to infections; the capacity to acknowledge and treat these health problems early is necessary for the successful survival paramedic. This section will certainly talk about several of the extra typical ones that you may see.

Different infections can create stomach pain, some of which can be treated clinically and also some which are dealt with surgically. One relatively typical concern that could be lethal in a long-term survival situation, especially to youngsters, would certainly be appendicitis. Appendicitis (swelling of the appendix) takes place in roughly 8 out of every 100 people. Appendicitis can take place in any individual; however, it probably influences individuals under 40. The appendix is a tubular worm-shaped item of tissue 2-4 inches long, which connects to the intestine at the reduced right side of the abdominal area. The inside of this structure forms a bag that available to the big intestinal tract. The appendix was once an important organ and remains in some animals (as an example, equines), but it is contracted and also nonfunctional in human beings. This is an instance of a "vestigial" organ, which suggests that it exists but serves a little helpful function.

The appendix causes trouble as a result of an obstruction. This allows microorganisms to multiply and also create inflammation, infection, and also fill up with pus. If the problem is not treated, the appendix can burst, spilling infected issue into the stomach caries. This triggers a problem called "peritonitis," which can spread out throughout the whole abdominal area and end up being extremely major. Before the growth of antibiotics, it was not uncommon to die from the infection; one popular sufferer was the silent film celebrity, Rudolph Valentino.

Some think that consuming a diet abundant in seeds is a reason for appendicitis. Others think that a lack of fiber in the diet plan causes smidgens of very difficult feces to come to be lodged in the organ. Although these are (rare) possibilities, the majority of instances have no evident cause. Appendicitis starts with obscure pain in the area of the stomach switch but relocates to the lower best quadrant of the abdomen after 12-24 hours.

Various other likely signs and symptoms might consist of:

- Queasiness as well as Throwing up
- Anorexia nervosa
- High temperature and also Chills
- Stomach Swelling
- Pain intensifying with coughs or strolling
- Difficulty passing gas
- Irregularity or Diarrhea

A person may resist using his legs, as that causes the movement of stomach muscles. Nausea, throwing up, and high temperature are various other typical symptoms and signs you may see. To detect this problem, push down on the lower right of the abdomen. Your patient will possibly find it agonizing. Continuing the left lower quadrant may generate pain in the lower right quadrant, as well. An indication of a feasible fractured appendix may be what is called "rebound tenderness." In this situation, weighing down will trigger pain, yet it will certainly be much more agonizing when you remove your hand. The client should be limited to small amounts of clear liquids as quickly as you make the medical diagnosis. Surgical elimination of the appendix is medicinal right here, yet it will certainly be challenging to accomplish without modern-day clinical centers.

If modern-day surgical treatment is unavailable, consider giving the patient prescription antibiotics by mouth in the hope of eliminating a very early infection. Of course, intravenous anti-biotics, such as Cefoxitin, are extra effective than associated oral antibiotics, such as Cephalexin (vet equivalent: Keflex or FISH-FLEX).

Researches in the UK accomplished some success utilizing intravenous anti-biotics in very early (uncomplicated) instances of appendicitis. A mix of Ciprofloxacin (veterinary equivalent: FISH-CIN), as well as Metronidazole (FISH-ZOLE), is an alternative if intravenous prescription antibiotics or surgical intervention is not available. It is additionally appropriate in that adverse Penicillin. Recuperation, although sluggish, may still be possible if therapy is started early enough or the body has created a wall surface around the infection. See the chapter on stockpiling drugs to learn more on anti-biotics.

Can the surgical procedure be performed in situations where the basic anesthetic is not available? A lot of surgical procedures can't, without the likelihood of shedding a patient. Having stated that, doctors in developing nations have, not uncommonly, done appendectomies under local anesthesia. Prior to surgery is considered to manage a swollen appendix, you must be particular that you are dealing with that specific trouble. In some cases, various medical problems present with similar signs and symptoms, as well as you will have to do some detective work to set apart one from an additional.

A few of infectious illness are as follows:

Urinary tract infection

Urinary tract infection is the name given to various inflammations of the mucous membrane of the urinary tract. These include those organs that transport the urine from the kidneys to the outside (ureter, bladder, and urethra). Most of the time, the bacteria rise from the urethra to the bladder and sometimes further towards the kidneys. Here you can read everything important about the different forms of urinary tract infection.

Mostly, a urinary tract infection is triggered by intestinal bacteria that pass from the anus into the outer urethra and then rise into the urogenital tract. Improper hygiene after using the toilet is often responsible for this. In other cases, urinary tract inflammation occurs after unprotected sexual intercourse. Women develop a urinary tract infection significantly more often. This is because women have a shorter urethra than men, which is why germs in them can get into the bladder more easily. Young women, in particular, are often affected by a urinary tract infection.

Children can also be affected by a urinary tract infection. There is an increased risk of infection, especially in diaper age, since bacteria can multiply rapidly in a moist environment. Other risk factors for urinary tract infections are a weakened immune system (e.g. due to serious illnesses or drugs suppressing the body's defense), metabolic disorders (such as diabetes mellitus), and urinary drainage disorder (e.g. due to urinary stones, tumors or enlarged prostate). Like most bacterial infections, urinary tract infection causes redness and swelling of the tissue. Typical urinary tract infection symptoms include pain and burning sensation during urination, blood in the urine, and a general feeling of illness. In severe cases, the urinary tract infection can also be accompanied by fever and chills. Many sufferers who repeatedly suffer from urinary tract infections recognize the first signs of a urinary tract infection early and can still avert impending cystitis with the help of home remedies.

Doctors distinguish between the so-called uncomplicated urinary tract infection from the complicated urinary tract infection. The doctor can usually diagnose "urinary tract infection" based on the typical symptoms and using a urine test strip. The test strip determines various typical changes in urine, such as the content of (parts of) red and white blood cells or certain products of the bacterial metabolism (nitrate).

In the case of complicated or frequently recurring urinary tract infections (medical: recurrent urinary tract infections), further diagnostics are necessary. For this purpose, so-called urine cultures are used to identify the bacteria responsible for the urinary tract infection and to test their sensitivity to antibiotic treatment. In such cases, bladder examinations (cystoscopy) can also be performed to discover previously unknown pathological changes in the urinary tract. The doctor can usually diagnose "urinary tract infection" based on the typical symptoms and using a urine test strip. The test strip determines various typical changes in urine, such as the content of (parts of) red and white blood cells or certain products of the bacterial metabolism (nitrate).

In the case of complicated or frequently recurring urinary tract infections (medical: recurrent urinary tract infections), further diagnostics are necessary. For this purpose, so-called urine cultures are used to identify the bacteria responsible for the urinary tract infection and to test their sensitivity to antibiotic treatment. In such cases, bladder examinations (cystoscopy) can also be performed to discover previously unknown pathological changes in the urinary tract.

Urinary tract infection therapy depends on the cause. A urinary tract infection can heal on its own, depending on the degree of expression and the body's immune system. If the body does not manage to fight urinary tract infection with its immune system, a doctor should be consulted immediately who will initiate appropriate treatment. Antibiotics are mostly used, which quickly and reliably bring about a reliable cure in the case of an uncomplicated urinary tract infection. The complicated urinary tract infection is also treated with antibiotics, but in this case the therapy takes longer.

Common liver infections

The liver is very resilient and can still do its job even if it is partially damaged. It can also repair damage very well as long as it is not too serious. However, if liver damage is recognized too late, it cannot be reversed. The liver itself does not contain any nerves, pressure pain under the right costal arch or upper abdominal cramps as a result of liver diseases arise rather from tension in the connective tissue capsule that envelops the liver. A typical side effect of liver diseases is fatigue and a drop in performance. This is why doctors also call "tiredness the pain of the liver." In addition, people with liver disease often suffer from impaired blood clotting because their liver is no longer able to produce the necessary proteins adequately. A blood test is an important tool for diagnosing liver diseases. If the liver is damaged, typical proteins from the cells get into the blood.

Hepatitis is inflammation/swelling of the liver. There are many causes of inflammation: viruses, bacteria, parasites or fungi, alcohol and other toxins, medicines, congenital disorders, radiation therapy, inflammation of the biliary tract, etc. The symptoms that hepatitis causes, how the disease develops, and how it is treated depend on the triggering cause. Typical symptoms of hepatitis are jaundice, fatigue, and sometimes itching. The primary biliary cirrhosis is a chronic inflammation of the biliary tract (cholangitis). The reason for this is unknown. Over 90% of the patients are women; mostly, they are older than 40 years. At first, there are few complaints, later itching, tiredness, poor performance, and indigestion. The disease cannot be cured; only its symptoms can be treated with medication. Primarily sclerosing cholangitis is an inflammation of the middle and larger bile ducts with an unknown cause. Up to 60% of patients have ulcerative colitis at the same time. The patients have itching and upper abdominal pain. Weight loss or jaundice may occur later. The disease cannot be cured; medication is given for the symptoms (e.g. itching). Bile duct cancer can result in the long term.

Cirrhosis of the liver is most often caused by constant excessive alcohol consumption or viruses caused by inflammation of the liver (hepatitis). In cirrhosis, the normal glandular tissue of the liver is rebuilt: nodules form, and the glandular tissue is replaced by connective tissue. The sinusoids and small vessels can, therefore, no longer remove blood. However, since blood continues to flow into the liver through the hepatic artery and portal vein, it builds up in front of the liver. This increases the pressure in the blood vessels, especially in the portal vein (portal vein pressure or portal hypertension). In addition, "advanced" liver cirrhosis can lead to jaundice.

The liver is an organ with multiple tasks. If she no longer works properly, this can have serious consequences for the entire body. In this information, you will learn more about the tasks of the liver, the meaning of the "liver values," and the most common liver diseases. You will receive tips on what you can do for a healthy liver yourself.

All cells need certain proteins for their own metabolism. The following are characteristic of the liver cells:

- Aspartate aminotransferase (AST)
- Alanine aminotransferase (ALT)
- Gamma Glutamyl Transferase (Gamma GT)
- Alkaline phosphatase (AP)

With liver damage, physical signs are usually very general, such as fatigue, tiredness, or feeling of pressure in the right upper abdomen. Many liver diseases are, therefore, not noticeable for a long time. Indicative signs such as yellowing of the eyes and skin, itching, vomiting, or pain often appear very late.

Inflammation of the liver can be triggered by various hepatitis viruses (A to E). The viruses are transmitted through food, feces, or body fluids such as blood. The inflammation usually heals on its own. However, sometimes it persists. Then drugs can help with hepatitis B and C.

Vaginal infection

Vaginal infections are caused by bacteria, fungi, viruses, or unicellular organisms; mixed infections are also possible. Typical symptoms are itching, burning, vaginal discharge, redness, swelling, and pain. The cause is usually a disturbed vaginal flora due to the decline in protective lactobacilli.

In fact, about 70% of women are regularly affected by infections in the genital area: uncomfortable burning, excruciating itching, or a foul-smelling discharge are usually not signs of poor hygiene, but often a clear indication of a vaginal infection. Vaginal infections are mainly caused by bacteria (40-50% of cases) or fungi (20-25%), viruses, or single-cell organisms (e.g. trichomonads) are less common. However, not only one type of pathogen is always responsible for the clinical picture: Often, one speaks of a mixed infection (bacteria and fungi can be found simultaneously, for example). Tight, non-absorbent underwear: With this underwear, moisture can accumulate, which facilitates infection by bacteria and fungi.

The natural vaginal flora of the healthy woman consists of a large number of different bacterial strains and is an essential protective shield against unpleasant infections. Numerous lactobacilli, which are also known as "Doderlein bacteria" after their discoverer, provide a slightly acidic environment in the vagina (pH 3.8 - 4.5), in which pathogenic germs can only reproduce with difficulty. All of these factors can easily upset the balance of the natural vaginal environment: important lactobacilli are then reduced and, as a result, unwanted microorganisms can colonize and multiply unhindered
The clinical symptoms of a vaginal infection are very diverse and, depending on the pathogen and depending on the female immune or hormone status, can be different, similar, or even completely absent. Special care should be taken with bacterial and fungal

infections, as they are often mistaken for one another without specialist advice.

The clinical symptoms of a vaginal infection are multifaceted and can be very different depending on the pathogen. For a reliable diagnosis, a thorough gynecological examination by the specialist is required: an uncomplicated swab from the vagina is carried out, which can then be examined microscopically. Most bacteria or fungi can be detected in this way.

In recurring or unclear cases, the smear is sent to a microbiological laboratory, where the exact pathogen (bacteria, fungi, viruses or unicellular organisms)
Vaginal infections can usually be treated with medication that works against individual pathogens (antibiotics against bacteria, antifungals against fungi, antivirals against viruses). Antiseptic agents (e.g. octenidine) work against a broad spectrum of pathogens, eliminate fungi and bacteria at the same time and are therefore an advantage for so-called mixed infections.

Attention: An unnecessary and incorrect use of antibiotics and antifungals harbors the risk of development of resistance of the pathogens involved, which makes sustainable therapy success even more difficult. Therefore, care should always be taken always to take prescribed antibiotics and antifungals exactly as directed by the treating doctor. Furthermore, taking antibiotics usually increases the risk of a subsequent yeast infection in the vagina.

Athlete's foot

Athlete's foot is the most common fungal infection; it is noticeable by itching and rash on the toes and feet. The athlete's foot is very contagious or very quickly infects other people or other parts of the body. Therefore it is essential to treat the fungus quickly. Here you can find out which different methods there are to get the problem with the fungus under control. Athlete's foot is a very common fungal infection, probably the most common of all. Young people and adults are particularly affected. Children are rarely affected by the fungus. People who actively exercise and often wear tight-fitting and non-breathable shoes are at particular risk of developing athlete's foot. The English expression for athlete's foot is "athlete's foot," although athletes are not the only ones who get athlete's foot.

The athlete's foot is also called "tenia pedis." And target the outmost skin of the foot. From here, it can spread to the skin between the other toes, the toenail, and possibly the entire foot. You will usually spot an athlete's foot due to the annoying itch that just won't go away. Between the toes, you can often see a reddish, slightly scaly rash. Sometimes there are small fluid-filled blisters between the toes.

Athlete's foot infects very easily, so it is extremely important to start treatment as soon as you realize you may have an athlete's foot. With immediate treatment, you can curb the infection so that it cannot spread to other parts of the body, and you don't infect others with the fungus. Athlete's foot is typically well hidden between the toes. Most of the time, the fungus begins to grow between the last and penultimate toe, and from there, it can spread to the other toes, nails, and feet.

The best thing you can do if you have the symptoms described is to see a doctor. The doctor can quickly diagnose whether it is an athlete's foot because a doctor is often confronted with this infection. It is extremely important to undergo immediate treatment so that the infection cannot spread to other parts of the body.
If the doctor has doubts, it may be necessary to scrape off some skin, which is then sent to a laboratory for further examination. It is no pain to scrape off some skin, and the whole thing is done very quickly. However, it may take a few weeks to get a result of the examination of the sample since the fungus has to be cultivated in the laboratory first, and unfortunately, this takes some time.

An infection causes athlete's foot with skin fungi, also called dermatophytes. It is a type of fungus that we all have in our bodies, just like many other fungi and bacteria that are native to our body and also live on our skin. Usually, the mushroom is completely harmless. It lives on dead skin cells and doesn't harm us. Athlete's foot is very contagious, so there is a possibility that someone else has given it to you. But there is also the possibility that you got athlete's foot without someone catching you or transmitting it to you. If your feet have been exposed to a warm and humid environment for a long time, the mushrooms have been given great conditions to grow or multiply. Fortunately, an athlete's foot is a completely harmless disease that is easy to treat. Both the treatment options and the effectiveness of the treatment are more than good. The most important thing is that you do not ignore the signs of a possible fungal disease. This could be difficult due to the itching.

Without treatment, you risk infecting others with your athlete's foot. But you also risk that the athlete's foot spreads to other parts of your body. For example, it can spread to the nails, which creates nail fungus. Nail fungus is much more difficult to cure than athlete's foot. See your doctor straight away if you think you have one or more fungi between your toes or feet.

If you don't do anything about an athlete's foot, you are not only risking it spreading and infecting someone. You also risk that the small cracks and wounds caused by athlete's foot give access to bacteria. If these bacteria penetrate the skin, you risk an infection like "erysipelas." Then it is no longer just a fungicidal treatment; then, it is also necessary to treat it with antibiotics.

Chapter 8

INJURIES

Your skin is considered an organ, indeed, the largest body organ in the body, and also serves as an obstacle versus infection and loss of fluids. When a burn deteriorates this obstacle, your health remains in jeopardy. Quick and also the efficient treatment of these injuries will avoid them from becoming deadly. Being the rugged individualists that they are, some in the preparedness or homesteading neighborhood may be most likely to disregard small injuries as insignificant. This couldn't be further from reality. Any small injury has the possibility to cause trouble later on. As a doctor throughout troubled times, you have to keep an eye on the recovery process of every wound. Each wound is various and has to be evaluated independently.

If not present at the time the wound is sustained, the medic should begin by asking the basic inquiry: "What happened"? A check out at the website of the mishap will certainly offer you a suggestion of what type of particles you may find in the injury and the likelihood of infection. Always presume an injury is filthy at first. The physical exam of an injury needs the adhering to analysis: Location on the body, length, depth, and also the sort of tissue entailed. Circulation and Nerve participation must likewise be reviewed. If an extremity, have the patient reveal you a full range of activity, preferably, during your assessment. This is especially crucial if the injury includes a joint. This section will certainly handle numerous injuries, their evaluation, and treatment. With close observation, your individuals will have the most effective opportunity of avoiding trouble.

Small injuries

A soft cell injury is taken into consideration minor when it fails to permeate the deep layer of the skin called the "dermis." This would certainly include cuts, scratches, and also wounds.

Cuts as well as Scratches: These tears in the skin only permeate the "epidermis" (superficial skin layer) and also end up being infected on a seldom basis in a healthy and balanced individual.

Abrasions or Scrapes: A part of the skin has been scraped off. You most likely have experienced a lot of these as a youngster. Contusions or Contusions: These result from blunt injury and also do not permeate the skin at all. Nevertheless, there is hemorrhaging into the skin from a capillary that has actually been interrupted by the impact.

Every one of the above minor injuries can be quickly treated. Wash the wound anywhere that the skin has been breached. The use of an antibacterial such as Betadine (Povidone-Iodine solution), honey, or three-way antibiotic lotion such as Neosporin or Bactroban will certainly be practical to stop the infection. Minor blood loss can be quit with a wet styptic pencil, and a product typically made use of for cutting cuts. The wound, if it broke the skin, must have a safety adhesive bandage (such as a Band-Aid) to avoid infection. Applying pressure and also ice (if available) and place a contusion appears to be spreading will stop it from growing. Bruises will certainly alter color with time from blackish-blue to brown to yellow.

The Fluid Skin plaster is an exceptional means to cover a small injury with some advantages over a normal plaster. You use it when to the cut or scrape; it dries out within a minute approximately as well as seals the injury. It also quits small blood loss, as well as won't befall throughout baths. There are numerous brands (Band-Aid Liquid Bandage, New Skin, Cured, 3M No Sting fluid plaster) and also many come as a practical spray. These injuries will certainly recover over the following 7-10 days, dependent on the quantity of skin area impacted.

You don't always need to take a trip to the standard roadway to deal with many clinical troubles. If you have among the minor injuries discussed, why not consider all-natural treatments? Below an alternate process to manage these concerns:

1. Review the severity of the wound; if minor, you may proceed with natural therapy.

2. Stop small bleeding with herbal blood clotting agents such as Chili pepper powder, as well as press the location with gauze. Materials that clot blood are called "hemostatic" representatives.

3. After minor blood loss is stopped, the injury ought to be cleansed with a natural antiseptic: Mix a couple of decreases of oil with clean and sterile water as well as wash out the injury completely.

4. Dress the wound using tidy gauze. Do not also wrap firmly.

5. Adjustment of the dressing reapplies antibacterial and also observes for infection two times daily up until healed.

Significant injuries

Cuts in the skin can be small or disastrous, superficial or deep, tidy, or infected. Many considerable cuts (likewise called 'lacerations') permeate both the dermis and epidermis and also are associated with bleeding, in some cases major. Recognizing exactly how to manage a hemorrhagic wound quickly as well as efficiently will be of paramount relevance. As the capillary, as well as the artery normally run together, a severe cut can have both. When below the level of the skin, big blood vessels, as well as nerves, might be entailed. Analyze blood circulation, experience, as well as the ability to relocate the hurt location. You will observe much more troubles with vessel and nerve damage in deep lacerations and also crush injuries.

For an extremity injury, review what we call the "Vein Refill Time" to check for flow past the location of the injury. To do this, press the nail bed or finger/toe pad; in an individual with the regular flow, this area will turn white when you launch pressure and then go back to a typical color within 2 seconds. If it takes longer or the fingertips are blue, you may have a person that has harmed a capillary. If electric motor feature or sensation is decreased (examination by lightly pricking with a safety pin past the degree of the injury), there might be nerve damages.

Assessing blood loss is a crucial facet of taking care of injuries. An ordinary dimension human grownup has around 10 pints of blood. The result of the body caused by blood loss varies with the amount of blood loss incurred:

- 1.5 pints (0.75 litres) or much less: little or no impact; you can donate a pint of whole blood, for example, as frequently as every eight weeks.

- 1.5-3.5 pints (0.75-1.5 litres): fast heartbeat and also respirations. The skin ends up being awesome and might show up light. The client is typically extremely flustered. If you are not accustomed to the sight of blood, you might also be. Even a percentage of blood on the floor or the individual might make an unskilled paramedic queasy.

- 3.5-4 pints (1.5-2 litres): High blood pressure starts to drop; the person may appear perplexed. Heartbeat is usually very quick.

- Over 4 pints (more than 2 litres): Patient is now extremely light, and also might be subconscious. After a time period with continued blood loss, the high blood pressure goes down, even more, the heart rate, as well as respirations reduce, and the patient remains in major danger.

When you come across an individual with a blood loss wound, the initial course of action is to quit the hemorrhage. Usually, direct pressure on the bleeding location may quit hemorrhaging all on its own. Bleeding in an extremity may be slowed by boosting the arm or leg above the level of the heart. The paramedic needs to have nitrile hand wear covers in his or her pack constantly; this will stop the wound from contamination by a "filthy" hand. Attempt to avoid touching the palm or finger portions of the hand wear covers as you put them on. If there are no gloves, grab a bandanna or various other cloth obstacles as well as press it right into the wound.

Furthermore, continuing the "pressure factor" for the area hurt may assist slow bleeding. Pressure points are areas where significant arteries come close sufficient to the skin to be compressed by hand. Continuing this area will certainly slow down hemorrhaging better down the track of the blood vessel? Making use of pressure factors, we can make a "map" of details locations to concentrate your efforts to reduce blood loss.

Soft cells injuries

As soon as you have actually quit the bleeding and also used your dressing, you are in safer territory than you were. In an ascetic set up, nonetheless, you must adhere to the standing of the wound until complete recovery in your function as a medic. Ongoing injury treatment is your obligation.

An open injury can heal by two techniques:

Key Intention (Closure): The injury is closed in some means, such as with stitches or staples. This results in a smaller sized scar but lugs the risk of unintentionally withdrawing microorganisms deep in the injury.

Additional Intention (Granulation): Leaving a wound open creates the development of "granulation tissue." Granulation tissue is rapidly growing, very early mark tissue that is rich in the capillary. It completes areas where the wound edges are not together. After a time period, it becomes mature scar tissue. This mark is larger than if the injury were nearby primary intent but decreased the danger of infection if effectively taken care of.
Typically, it is most safe to allow a wound to heal by itself rather than stitch or staple it closed. Wound dressings must be changed regularly (at the very least twice a day or whenever the bandage is filled with blood, liquids, etc.) in order to provide the most effective chance for quick recovery. When you alter a dressing, it is necessary to clean up the wound location with drinkable water.

Remember the old saying, "The remedy to air pollution is dilution." Making use of a bulb or irrigation syringe (60-100 ml) will certainly give pressure to the flow of water and also wash out old clots and dirt. Gently scrub any kind of open injury with watered-down Betadine or disinfected water. You might observe some (usually slight) blood loss. This suggests cells that are forming new blood vessels, as well as not always a poor indicator. Apply pressure with a tidy bandage up until it stops. Remarkably, a lot of studies discover that sanitized (drinkable) water is equally as good as a focused antiseptic solution for wound recovery (in some cases far better). Although it is acceptable to perform a very first cleaning with Betadine or Hydrogen Peroxide, later cleaning must most definitely not utilize these concentrated items. New cells are trying to grow, and also they do this ideal in a damp atmosphere. Concentrated antiseptics dry out these delicate brand-new cells as well as make reduce healing.

Burn injuries

If you cannot avoid extensive exposure to sunshine, be specific to use a sunscreen. They ought to be applied prior to going outside and also regularly throughout the day. Even water-resistant/proof sun blocks need to be reapplied every 1-2 hrs. Most individuals fail to put enough on their skin; be generous in your application.

By the way, a sunblock and also a sunblock are not the very same thing. Sunblock includes tiny particles that "block" as well as reflect UV light. A sunscreen has substances that take in UV light, thus avoiding it from passing through the skin. Lots of business products have both. The SPF (Sun Protection Aspect) rating system was established in 1962 to measure the capacity of an item to obstruct UV radiation. It determines the size of time your skin will certainly be secured from burning.

An SPF (sunlight defense element) of a minimum of 15 is suggested. It takes about 20 mins without sunblock for your skin to turn red. A product that is SPF 15 must delay burning by an element of 15, or concerning 5 hrs.' or so. Greater SPF scores provide even more security, as well as could be beneficial to those with fair skin.

Besides the sunlight, injuries will certainly most likely be associated with food preparation, especially by the campfire. Making use of hand security will certainly avoid many of these burns, as will mindful supervision of kids near any kind of cooking area. Now, allow concentrate on discovering to recognize burns by their level:

First Degree Burns

These burns will be really common, such as simple sunburn. The injury will certainly show up red, warm as well as dry, as well as will certainly be painful to the touch. These burns frequently impact large locations of the upper body; immersion in a great bathroom is a good idea or a minimum of running amazing water over the injury.
Putting an amazing moist towel or Spenco will certainly give some relief. As Ibuprofen also gives relief because it has anti-inflammatory properties.

Aloe Vera or Zinc Oxide cream is additionally an efficient therapy. Normally, the discomfort enhances after 24-hour or so, as only the surface skin layer, the skin, is influenced. Avoid tight clothing and also try to put on light materials, such as cotton.

Second-Degree Burns

These burns are deeper, going partly via the skin, and also will certainly be seen to be wet and have sores with reddened bases. The area will have a tendency to weep clear or creamy colored fluid. The location will appear slightly puffy, so eliminate rings and also bracelets.

To treat 2nd degrees burns:

· Run awesome water over the injury for 10-15 minutes (stay clear of ice).
· Apply wet skin dressings such as Spenco Second skin.
· Give oral discomfort relief such as Ibuprofen.
· Apply anesthetic ointment such as Benzocaine. Use Silver Sulfadiazine (Silvadene) lotions to aid prevent infection.
· Consider antibiotic lotion if slow-moving to heal.
· Lance only large sores
· Stay clear of eliminating burnt skin.

A personal apart: I had a substantial second level burn as a kid (they called it "sunlight poisoning" back then), and my little sibling thought it was a great idea to peel some skin. It does not peel off the skin from a second level burn.

Third-Degree Burns

The awful kind of burn injury; it includes the complete thickness of skin and possibly much deeper frameworks such as subcutaneous fat and also muscular tissue. It may show up charred, or be white in the shade. The shed may show up indented if substantial tissue has actually been lost. Third-degree burns will certainly create dehydration, so giving liquids is necessary to keep the patient stable. Spenco Second Skin is, once more, beneficial, as a burn injury cover, for security purposes.
Celox combat gauze, when wet, creates a gel-like dressing that may provide a handy obstacle. Silver Sulfadiazine (Silvadene) lotion is useful in avoiding infections in third-degree burns.

They would certainly be dealt with the same as third-degree burns in a lasting survival situation. Any melt this serious that is larger than, state, an inch or two in size, usually needs a skin graft to heal entirely. Regrettably, the capacity for such restorative surgery is unlikely to be readily available. An individual with third-degree burns over more than 10% of the body surface could be going into shock and remains in a life-endangering situation.

When a person obtains shed, it's of paramount relevance to eliminate the warm resource right away. Run cool water over any type of level of the shed for at the very least 10-15 minutes ASAP after the injury. Awesome water is more suitable to ice as it is less terrible to the currently damaged tissue. Once again, be particular to eliminate rings or fashion jewelry, as swelling is frequently seen in these sorts of injuries.

Head injuries

Head injuries can be soft tissue injuries (mind, scalp, blood vessels) or bony injuries (head, facial bones), so I've placed this section between soft tissue as well as orthopedic issues. Damage is normally triggered by straight effects, such as a laceration in the scalp or a fracture of the part of the head, which contains the brain (also called the "cranium").

An "open" head injury means that the head has actually been permeated with possible direct exposure of the brain cells. If the head is not fractured, it is referred to as a "closed" injury. Damage can also be brought on by the rebound of the mind versus the inside wall surfaces of the skull; this might create tearing of the blood vessels in mind, which can cause a hemorrhage. There may be no noticeable permeating injury in this situation; the initial trauma may even have occurred at a website besides the head. An example of this would certainly be the fierce trembling of an infant.

Anybody with a traumatic injury to the head should always be observed very closely, as signs and symptoms from bleeding as well as swelling might take time to establish. The brain needs blood as well as oxygen to function typically. An injury that causes bleeding or swelling inside the skull will raise intracranial stress. This triggers the heart to function more difficult to obtain blood and oxygen right into the mind. Blood build-up (known as a "hematoma") can happen within the mind cells, itself, or from in between the layers of tissue covering the brain. Without sufficient circulation, mind function stops.

Stress that is high enough might actually create a portion of the brain to push downward with the base of the skull. This is called a "brain herniation," as well as, without modern medical care, will nearly inevitably lead to fatality. The majority of head injuries cause only a laceration to the scalp and also a swelling at the site of impact. Cuts on the scalp or face will certainly tend to bleed, as numerous small blood vessels take a trip with this location. This blood loss, although substantial, does not have to symbolize interior damage; most instances can be treated as any other laceration. There are a variety of symptoms and signs, however, which may recognize those individuals that are a lot more severely affected. They consist of:

- Loss of Awareness
- Convulsions (Seizures)
- Worsening Headache
- Nausea or vomiting, as well as Vomiting
- Discoloration (around eyes as well as ears)
- Bleeding from Ears and also Nose
- Confusion/Apathy/Drowsiness

Indentation of the Head

An individual with trauma to the head may be knocked unfamiliarity for an amount of time or may stay completely alert. If awareness is not shed, the individual may experience a headache and might call for treatment for surface injuries. After a duration of observation, a head injury without loss of consciousness is more than likely not serious unless among the various other symptoms and signs from the above checklist are kept in mind.

Loss of awareness for a very quick time (claim, 2 minutes or so) will merit close observation for the following two days. A head injury of this kind is called a "concussion." This client will generally stir up somewhat "foggy," and also might be uncertain regarding exactly how the injury happened or the occasions quickly before. It will be essential to be specific that the person has restored regular motor function. Simply put, see to it they can move all their extremities with typical array and also toughness. Even so, rest is recommended for the remainder of the day, so that they might be carefully enjoyed.

When your individual is asleep, it will be appropriate to awaken them every 2-3 hours, to make certain that they are conveniently excited and have created none of the danger signals noted above. For the most part, a concussion triggers no permanent damage unless there are multiple episodes of head injury gradually, as in the case of fighters or other professional athletes.

If the duration of unconsciousness is over 10 minutes in size, you should think about the possibility of significant injury. Essential indicators such as pulse, respiration rate, and also high blood pressure ought to be monitored very closely. The individual's head needs to be incapacitated, and focus needs to be offered to the neck and spine, in case they are additionally damaged. Confirm that the respiratory tract is clear, and also get rid of any kind of possible blockages. In a collapse, he or she is in a serious circumstance that will have a couple of medicinal options if awareness is not gained back.

Other signs of a significant injury to this location are the appearance of wounding behind the ears or around the eyes (the "raccoon" indicator) in spite of the impact not occurring in that area. This could suggest a crack with interior blood loss. Bleeding from the ear itself or nose without straight injury to those locations is another indication. The liquid might be clear and not bloody; this might stand for spine liquid leak.
Furthermore, intracranial blood loss might trigger stress that presses nerves that cause the pupils. In this case, you will certainly discover that your subconscious client has one student more dilated than the various others.

A stroke (also known as a cerebrovascular accident or CVA) is damage to the brain brought on by a lack of blood supply. This might occur in a head injury because of a blockage of blood to a part of the mind. This clog

could be due to a clot, a hemorrhage, or anything else that endangers the flow in the area. Whatever functions are related to the part of the mind influenced will certainly be shed or harmed. This could consist of
the failure to speak, blindness, or loss of normal understanding. Signs, such as paralysis or weak point, are typically on one side of the body and face. An abrupt serious frustration usually proclaims the stroke.

Strokes might take place due to other reasons as well, such as unchecked hypertension. Although it may not be hard to detect a significant CVA in an austere setting, few options will exist for treating it. Blood slimmer's could aid a stroke triggered by an embolism, yet intensify a stroke caused by hemorrhage. Maybe hard to inform, which is without innovative screening? Maintain the target on bed remainder; often, they may recuperate partial feature after an amount of time. If they do, a lot of renovation will happen in the first couple of days.

Chapter 9

ANIMAL BITES

Most individuals have, at some time of their life, run afoul of an ornery pet dog or pet cat. Many pet attacks will certainly be puncture injuries; these will certainly be reasonably small but have the potential to cause dangerous infections. In the United States, there are millions of pet attacks annually. Many pet attacks influence the hands (in grownups) and the face, head, and also neck (in kids). Residential animals, such as felines, dogs, as well as tiny rats, are the culprits in the grand majority of situations. Pet dog attacks, the most common, are generally extra shallow than pet cat attacks, as their teeth are reasonably plain contrasted to felines. Despite this, their jaws are powerful as well as can inflict crush injuries to soft tissues. Cats' teeth are thin and sharp, and leak wounds often tend to be much deeper. Both can bring about infection if neglected. However, cat bites inject bacteria right into deeper tissues and appear to end up being contaminated more frequently.

Besides the injury related to the actual bite, numerous pets bring condition which can be sent to people. Right

here are just a couple of illness as well as the pets included:
Rabies: Viral diseases spread out by raccoons, skunks, bats, opossums, and also dogs. Plague: Microbial condition associated with rats as well as fleas.

Consumption: Bacterial condition associated with deer, elk, and also bison.
Brucella: Bacterial disease related to bison, deer, and also other pets. Hantavirus: Viral illness brought on by computer mice. Baylisascaris (raccoon roundworm): Parasitical illness connected with raccoons.

Histoplasma: Fungal disease associated with bat excrement (guano).

Tularemia: Microbial illness connected with wildlife, especially rats, bunnies, and hares.
Additionally, it is possible to develop tetanus from any animal bite. Tetanus is a possibly fatal infection of the muscles as well as nerves triggered by the bacteria Clostridia.

Individuals who removed their spleen

Whenever an individual has been attacked, the initial, as well as the most important activity, is to put on hand wear covers and tidy the injury extensively with soap as well as water. Purging the wound with an irrigation syringe will certainly help eliminate dust as well as bacteria-containing saliva. Benzalkonium Chloride (BZK) is the best antiseptic to utilize in dealing with pet bites, due to the fact that it has some effect versus the Rabies virus. Make sure to manage any kind of blood loss with straight pressure (for more details, see the section on hemorrhagic wounds).

Any animal bite ought to be thought about a "dirty" wound as well as must not be taped, sutured, or stapled shut. If the bite is on the hand, any type of rings or bracelets need to be taken off; if swelling happens, they might be very tough to get rid of later on. Frequent cleaning is the most effective therapy for a recuperating bite wound. Apply antibiotic ointment to the location and also make certain to expect indicators of infection. You may see soreness, swelling, or oozing. In lots of circumstances, the site could feel abnormally warm to the touch.

Dental antibiotics might be appropriate therapy (specifically after a cat bite): Clindamycin (veterinary matching: Fish-Cin) 300mg by mouth every 6 hours and also. Ciprofloxacin (Fish-Flox) 500 mg every 12 hrs. in the mix would certainly be a great option. However, Azithromycin, as well as Ampicillin-Sulbactam, are also options. A tetanus shot is shown in those who have not been immunized in the last five years. Youngsters who endure pet attacks might establish a form of Post-traumatic Stress Syndrome (discussed later on in this publication) from experience and might call for therapy.

The grand majority of situations are found in underdeveloped countries. In the United Kingdom, rabies is almost uncommon, although there has actually been a report or two of infection from bat attacks in 2012. Although the timeless example is the rabid pet, pet cat bites are one of the most typical causes among domesticated animals. Wild animals, nonetheless, accounts for the grand bulk of situations in the USA.

Raccoons, opossums, skunks, coyotes, as well as bats are the most common vectors.

A person with rabies is generally symptom-free temporarily, which differs in each instance (ordinary 30 days or so). The person will certainly start to experience fatigue, high temperature, migraine, loss of appetite, and fatigue. The site of the bite injury might be itchy or numb. A couple of days later on, evidence of nerve damages shows up in the form of irritability, disorientation, hallucination, seizures, and, ultimately, paralysis. The sufferer might go into a coma or endure cardiac or breathing apprehension.

When an individual develops the illness, it is normally fatal

Inoculations are readily available to prevent the condition. Regardless of your general viewpoint regarding them, it might be something to consider (specifically if you function with pets as an occupation). It is necessary to remember that human beings are pets, and you could see attacks from this resource also. About 10-15% of human attacks become contaminated due to the truth that there are over 100 million microorganisms per milliliter in saliva.

Although it would certainly be astonishingly rare to obtain rabies as a result of a human bite, transmission of hepatitis, tetanus, herpes, syphilis, and also HIV when possible, deal with as you would any type of infected wound. Be specifically specific not to shut slit injuries from bites, as they would likely become infected if you do.

Snake bite

Poisons and also poisonous substances are not the same point. Poisonous substances are soaked up by the skin or digestion system, but poisons need to go into the cells or blood straight. For that reason, it is usually not hazardous to consume alcohol snake poison unless you have, state, a cut in your mouth (do not try it, though). The United States and Canada have two kinds of poisonous snakes: The pit vipers (rattlesnakes, water moccasins) and also Elapids (reefs snakes). Several of these snakes can be discovered nearly everywhere in the continental U.S.A participant of additional viper family members, the usual adder, is the only poisonous snake in Britain. However, it and also various other adders are common throughout Europe (besides Ireland, thanks to St. Patrick).

These snakes normally have hollow fangs through which they supply venom. Snakes are most energetic during the warmer months, and also, for that reason, most attack injuries are seen then. Not every bite from a poisonous snake transfers its poisonous substance to the sufferer; 25-30% of these attacks will reveal no ill effects. This probably concerns the period of time the snake has its fangs in its victim. An ounce of avoidance, they say, is worth a pound of cure. Make certain to wear excellent solid high-top boots and long pants when hiking in the wild. Stepping greatly develops ground vibrations and noise, which will certainly frequently cause snakes to hit the road. Snakes have no outer ear, so they "hear" ground vibrations far better than those in the air brought on by, for example, yelling.

Numerous snakes are active in the evening, particularly in cozy weather conditions. Some tasks of daily survival, such as gathering firewood, are advisable with a good light. In the wild, it is necessary to look where you're putting your hands and also feet. Be specifically careful around locations where snakes might such as to conceal, such as hollow logs, under rocks, or in old shelters. Using heavy gloves would be a sensible precaution.

A snake does not constantly wriggle away after it attacks you. It's most likely that it still has more venom that it can infuse, so vacate its region or eliminate the threat whatsoever you can. Killing the snake, nonetheless, might not make it harmless: it can reflexively bite for a time period, even if its head has been cut from its body. Snake bites that trigger a burning pain immediately are most likely to have poison in them. Swelling at the website may begin as quickly as 5 minutes afterward, and may take a trip up the damaged area. Pit viper bites tend to cause discoloration and also blisters at the site of the wound. Pins and needles may be kept in mind in the area bitten, or perhaps on the lips or face. Some targets describe a metallic or other odd preference in their mouths.

With pit vipers, wounding is not unusual as well as a serious bite might begin to cause spontaneous blood loss from the nose or gum tissues. Coral reefs snake attacks, however, will certainly cause mental and nerve issues such as twitching, complication as well as slurred speech. Later on, nerve damages might trigger a problem with ingesting and breathing, complied with by total paralysis. Reefs snakes show up very comparable to their look-alike, the non-venomous king snake. They have red, yellow, and also black bands, as well as are generally puzzled with each other. The old stating goes:

"red touches yellow, kill a fellow; red touches black, venom it lacks." This adage only puts on coral snakes in North America, nevertheless.

The treatment for a poisonous snake bite is "Antivenin," an animal or human serum with antibodies with the ability to reduce the effects of a certain biological contaminant. This item will most likely not be available in a lasting survival scenario.

The following strategy, as a result, will be useful:

- Keep the target calm. Stress and anxiety raise blood flow, therefore endangering the client by speeding the poison right into the system.

- Quit all motion of the hurt extremity. Activity will relocate the poison into the flow much faster, so do your ideal to keep the arm or leg still.

- Tidy the wound thoroughly to get rid of any type of poison that isn't deep in the wound, and get rid of rings and bracelets from a damaged extremity. Swelling is most likely to take place. Setting the extremity below the degree of the heart; this additionally reduces the transport of poison. Wrap with compression bandages as you would certainly an orthopedic injury, but continue it better up the limb than typical. Wrapping begins two to four inches over the bite (towards the heart), winding around as well as moving up, then pull back over the bite as well as past it towards the hand or foot.

- Maintain the covering about as limited as to when dressing a sprained ankle. If it is too limited, the person will reflexively relocate the limb, and move the poison around.

- Do not make use of tourniquets, which will certainly do more harm than excellent.

Draw a circle, when possible, around the affected location. As time progresses, you will certainly see enhancement or intensifying at the site much more clearly. This is a useful strategy to follow any kind of local response or infection. The arm or leg must then be relaxed and possibly debilitated with a splint or sling. The much less movement there is, the far better. Keep the person on bed remainder, with the bite website lower than the heart for 24-48 hrs. This strategy additionally benefits bites from poisonous reptiles, like Gila monsters. It is no longer suggested to make a laceration and try to suck out the poison with your mouth. If done greater than 3 minutes after the real bite, it would certainly remove maybe 1/1000 of the poison and could cause damage or infection to the bitten location. A Sawyer Extractor (a syringe with a suction cup) is much more modern. However, it is also relatively inefficient in getting rid of more than a percentage of the venom. These techniques stop working, mainly, as a result of the rate at which the poison is taken in.

Insects bite as well as stings

The exemptions are black widow crawlers, brown hermit crawlers, and also various caterpillars and also scorpions. A number of these attacks can infuse toxins that might trigger significant damages. Naturally, we are discussing the bite itself, not a condition that may be passed on by the pest. We will discuss that topic in the section on the mosquito-borne disease.

Bee/Wasp Stings

Stinging bugs can be inconveniences; however, for up to 3% of the population, they can be serious. In the USA, 40-50 fatalities a year are triggered by hypersensitivity responses. For most targets, the transgressor will be a bee, wasp, or hornet. A bee will certainly leave its stinger in the target, but wasps take their stingers with them and can sting once more. Even though you won't obtain hurt once again by the same bee, they send out an aroma that informs nearby bees that an assault is underway. This is particularly real with Africanized bees, which are much more hostile than indigenous bees. Because of this, you must leave the location whether the wrongdoer was a wasp or hornet.

The best method to lower any reaction to venom is to eliminate the stinger as quickly as feasible. Pull it out with tweezers or, preferably, scuff it out with your fingernail. The poison cavity of a need to not be adjusted as it will undoubtedly infuse extra irritant right into the sufferer. Many bee and wasp stings recover with little or no therapy. For those that experience just neighborhood reactions, complying with actions will certainly enough.

Get rid of the stinger if visible

Place cold packs as well as anesthetic lotions to ease the pain as well as regional swelling—control itching as well as inflammation with dental antihistamines such as

Benadryl or Claritin. Offer Acetaminophen or ibuprofen to reduce discomfort.

Apply antibiotic ointments to prevent infection

Some scorpions may reach a number of inches long; they have eight legs and also pincers, and infuse venom through their "tail." They are most typically active at night. Interestingly, scorpion exoskeletons somewhat fluorescent under ultraviolet light; you can locate them most quickly at night by using a "black light." A scorpion sting most often influences the nervous system. Youngsters are most in jeopardy for major complications. Signs you may see in victims of scorpion stings might include:

- Discomfort, numbness, and tingling in the location of the sting
- Sweating
- Weakness
- Boosted saliva output
- Restlessness or twitching
- Irritability
- Trouble ingesting
- Quick breathing and heart price

When you have actually identified a scorpion sting, do the following:
Wash the area with soap as well as water. Eliminate fashion jewelry from an impacted arm or leg (swelling might occur). Apply cool compresses to reduce pain. Offer an antihistamine, such as diphenhydramine (Benadryl). If done swiftly, this may slow down the poison's spread. Keep your individual calm to decrease the spread of venom. Limit food consumption if the

throat is swollen. Provide pain relievers such as Ibuprofen. Acetaminophen, yet stays clear of narcotics, as they might suppress breathing. Do not cut in the injury or usage suction to try to get rid of the poison. Although not likely available in an austere setting, an antivenin is currently readily available that gets rid of signs in children (the team most badly affected) after 4 hrs.

Fire Ant Bites

Fire ants are about 1/4 inch in length and also can be red or black. If their nest is disturbed, it causes a mass attack of, sometimes, thousands of nest participants. The ants bite with their jaws as well as have a rear-end stinger that they can make use of several times. Hypersensitivity to fire ants triggers concerning 80 fatalities a year in the Southeastern USA. If fire ants strike you, do the following:

- Brush them away with your hands (although it might be tough if they have secured their jaws into you).
- Relocate away from the pile.
- Remove clothing if they may have entered them.
- Raise the bitten extremity to decrease swelling.
- Area a cool compress on the location.
- If a blister establishes, do not pop it. It will usually not get contaminated if it stays intact.
- If sore pops, wash with soap and water. Think about anti-biotics, such as Amoxicillin, if the wounds appear to worsen with time.

Bedbugs

Of all the creepy-crawlies that raise an alarm system in a household, a couple of are even worse than bed insects. Although the bad standard of lives, as well as unsanitary conditions, have actually been associated with bed bug infestations, even the cleanest house in one of the most developed nations can harbor these parasites.

Bed bugs were as soon as so typical that every home in several urban locations was thought to nurture them in the early 20th century. They declined with the arrival of contemporary pesticides like DDT. Still, a revival of these creatures has actually been noted in The United States and Canada, Europe, and also Australia over the last decade or so. Cities such as New York and London have actually seen five times as numerous instances reported over the last couple of years. This may have to do with the limitation of DDT-like pesticides. On the other hand, the basic over-use of chemicals might be causing resistance.

The typical bed bug (Cimex Lectularius) is a little wingless bug that is thought to have actually come from caverns where both bats, as well as humans, made their residences. Ancient Greeks, such as Aristotle, discuss them in their writings. They were such a major concern throughout WWII that Zyklon, a Hydrogen Cyanide gas infamously utilized in Nazi concentration camps, was applied by both sides to eliminate invasions.

There are a variety of species of bed insects that are discovered in varying climates. Unlike lice, bed pests are not constantly species-specific (special to human beings). As an example, Cimex hemipterus, a bed bug discovered in tropical regions infests poultry and bats as well as people.

Adult bed bugs are light to tool brownish as well as have an oval, level bodies regarding 4mm lengthy (a little more after eating). Juveniles are called "fairies" as well as are lighter in the shade, nearly transparent. There are numerous fairy stages before adulthood; to proceed to the adult years, a dish of blood (yours!) is needed.

Bed bugs, which are mainly (yet not specifically) energetic at night, bite the exposed skin of resting human beings to eat their blood; they then retreat to concealing areas in joints of the bed mattress, linens, as well as furniture. Their attacks are typically painless, but later on, itchy elevated welts on the skin might establish. The extent of the action varies from one person to another.

Chapter 10

EPIDEMICS AND VIRUSES

An epidemic is a break out of global percentages. It occurs when a bacteria or unique infection ends up being effective in spreading out rapidly. It triggers major diseases in addition to can spread out conveniently from a bachelor to the complying with. Words pandemic originates from the Greek word suggesting "concerning all individuals. Everyone should know the essential first aid measures. But be careful. The theory is not the only thing that matters. Only if you regularly train the life-saving handles yourself will they be easy and safe to handle in an emergency! That is why this book recommended. Refresh your first aid knowledge at least every three years with training or a new course.

Quick realities on upsurges and infections

- Epidemics are typically brought on by a novel transmittable agent, a transmittable representative that is new with the ability to expand quickly, or both.

- The death toll in a pandemic is generally higher than that in an epidemic.

- The Spanish flu was the most terrible pandemic in the background, removing 100 million people.
- Boosted travelling as well as likewise, adaptability has actually increased the opportunity of new problems spreading out.

- Antibiotic resistance boosts the risk of future pandemics.

Pandemic or epidemic

The casualty of a pandemic is normally much higher than that of an epidemic. A pandemic is when a disease spreads throughout a vast geographical place and also influences lots of people. An epidemic is specific to one city, area, or nation, yet a pandemic spreads past nationwide boundaries, potentially worldwide. A native illness is one that continuously exists in a specific location or location. An epidemic is when the range of individuals that experience an infection is greater than the number expected within a nation or a part of a nation. If an infection winds up being substantial in numerous nations at the same time, it can end up being a pandemic. A pandemic is usually induced by new infection stress or subtype that becomes quickly transmissible in between people, or by bacteria that happen unsusceptible to antibiotic therapy. In some cases, pandemics are produced simply by a new ability to spread out swiftly, such as with the Black Death. Human beings could have little or no resistance against a brand-new infection.

Regularly a new infection cannot expand in between people; nevertheless, if it alters or mutates, it might begin to spread out rapidly. In this circumstance, a pandemic can result. In the case of influenza (influenza), seasonal episodes or booms-- are commonly activated by subtypes of an infection that is currently distributing among individuals. Pandemics, on the other hand, are generally triggered by novel subtypes. These subtypes have actually not dispersed among people prior to. Pandemic influences even more individuals, as well as can be much more deadly than an epidemic. It can furthermore bring about a lot more social disruption, financial loss, in addition to the basic challenge.

Influenza epidemics

A pandemic can take place when a type of flu infection, known as the flu, an infection, changes all of a sudden. This change can cause an infection that is different than any type of infection that currently exists. On the surface of the infection are HA healthy and balanced proteins and NA healthy and balanced proteins. If one or both of this adjustment, brand-new influenza An infection subtype can result. If this subtype obtains the capacity to spread out in between people, a pandemic can result. After the epidemic emerges and additionally spreads out, human beings create some resistance. After that, the infection subtype can distribute amongst people for many years, creating periodic flu upsurges. Various bodies worldwide, such as the Globe Health Company as well as the Centers for Health Problem Control and also Evasion (CDC) watch on the actions and likewise activities of the infection.

Background

The Spanish flu pandemic, from 1918 to 1920, asserted 100 million lives. It is taken into consideration the most awful in history. The Black Death asserted the lives of over 75 million individuals in the 14th Century. Some pandemics, as well as upswings that have actually occurred, include:

The Black Fatality eliminated 30-60% of Europe's complete populace.

- Plague of Justinian 541.
- Black Fatality 1346-1350.
- Cholera 1899-1923.
- Spanish influenza (H1N1) 1918-1920.
- Eastern influenza (H2N2) 1957-1958.
- Hong Kong flu 1968-1969.
- Bird influenza (H1N1) 2009.

Some infections exist in pet dogs, however rarely infected humans. Sometimes an event can happen that makes this possible. Wellness and wellness authorities are worried when an instance arises of a pet virus passing to humans, as this can be an indicator that the infection is altering. Swine influenza and bird-- or avian-- influenza, describe infections that prevailed in pigs or birds, however not in individuals, till an antigenic change took place. In recent times, there has likewise been a problem with infections that have been connected to camels (creating Middle East Respiratory Disorder, or MERS) and likewise apes (Ebola).

Stages

The etiology of upsurges can be separated right into six stages. There is a six-stage influenza program:

Stage 1

No family pet flu virus dispersing amongst animals has, in fact, been reported to activate infection in people.

Stage 2

A pet flu infection circulating in domesticated or wild animals is recognized to have triggered infection in people, in addition, to be consequently thought about an information possible pandemic danger.

Stage 3

Human-animal influenza reasserting infection has really developed occasional scenarios or little collections of the problem in individuals. Yet, it has actually not caused human-to-human transmission enough to obtain community-level breakouts.

Stage 4

Human-to-human transmission of an animal or human-animal influenza reasserting infection able to maintain community-level episodes has really been validated.

Stage 5

A similar well-known infection has actually produced sustained area level outbreaks in two or more countries.

Stage 6

In addition to the standards defined in Stage 5, the precise very same infection has created continual area level episodes in a minimum of another country in an additional that region.

Post-peak duration

A degree of pandemic influenza in most countries with appropriate tracking has, in fact, dropped listed below peak degrees.

Post-epidemic duration

Levels of flu activity have actually gone back to the degrees seen for seasonal flu in a lot of nations with adequate tracking.

Modern upsurges

If an influenza pandemic were to emerge today, the adhering to problems could arise. Individuals today are a lot more globally mobile and more than likely to remain in cities than in the past, variables that increase the threat of an infection dispersing. Faster interaction increases the danger of panic, as well as additionally the possibility that individuals that might be infected will certainly take a trip in an effort to get away the illness, potentially taking the infection with them. It can take months or years for vaccination to show up since pandemic viruses are one-of-a-kind representatives. Professional facilities would definitely be bewildered, in addition to there could be deficiencies of employees to give crucial community service, as a result of both the demand as well as additionally ailment.

The complying with is all feasible origin of worry:

- Viral hemorrhagic heats.
- Viral hemorrhagic fevers, including the Ebola and likewise Marburg viruses, might become pandemics.
- Nevertheless, a close call is needed for these conditions to spread.

Modern monitoring systems, lessons got from the Ebola episode in West Africa in 2014 to 2015, and also a speculative injection that is currently readily available for individuals that could be affected by the condition, make use of hope that, in future, brand-new circumstances will certainly be managed promptly which the condition can be consisted of.

Flu

Wild birds are a natural host for a selection of influenza stress. In unusual situations, these influenza varieties can pass from bird to human, setting off upsurges with the prospective to develop into pandemics, if left uncontrolled. Bird flu (H5N1) is an instance of this. The tension was first acknowledged in Vietnam in 2004. It never ever
reached epidemic levels, yet the feasible capability of the infection to incorporate with human influenza infections is a worry to researchers.

Ebola

The largest Ebola epidemic the world has really ever seen affected Liberia in addition to surrounding nations in West Africa in 2014 to 2015. Massive initiatives to have the problem prevented it from coming to be a pandemic. Ebola has really just recently resurfaced in the Democratic Republic of Congo, in Central Africa, along with that is inspecting the scenario.

The Most Damaging upsurges.

As drug developments, there are less contagious ailment episodes or epidemics. An epidemic is when a contagious ailment spreads within a location or area throughout a certain period. Discover the biggest episodes to spread out throughout the United States, and likewise where we are now.

1633-1634: Smallpox from European inhabitants.

Smallpox concerned The United States and also Canada in the 1600s. People had signs of high fever, cools, extreme discomfort in the back, in addition to rashes. Beginning with the Northeast, smallpox eliminated whole Native American people. Over 70 percent of the Aboriginal American population went down. In 1721, 844 of the 5,889 Bostonians that had smallpox died from it.

End: In 1770, Edward Jenner produced a vaccination from cowpox. It helps the body become unsusceptible to smallpox without triggering the disease.

Presently: After a big vaccination initiative in 1972, smallpox is gone from the UNITED STATES. As a matter of fact, inoculations are no more needed.

1793: Yellow fever from the Caribbean

Philly was as soon as the country's sources, along with its busiest port. One moist summertime season, refugees leaving a yellow fever epidemic in the Caribbean Islands travelled in, bring the infection with them. Yellow high temperature develops yellowing of the skin, heat, and also bloody throwing up. Five thousand individuals passed away, as well as 17,000 left the city.

End: The injection was developed and afterward accredited in 1953. One vaccination is completely enough. It's mostly recommended for those nine months and also older, particularly if you live or take a trip to dangerous locations. You can discover these particular nations at the Centers for Condition Control and also Avoidance (CDC) website.

Now: Mosquitoes are vital to how this condition spreads, particularly in nations like Central as well as South America as well as Africa. Eliminating them has actually succeeded in controlling yellow high temperature. While yellow high temperature has no treatment, someone that does recover from the illness becomes immune for the remainder of their life.

1832-1866: Cholera in 3 waves

The United States had three major waves of cholera, somehow between 1832 and 1866. The pandemic began in India and quickly spread across the globe through trade routes. New York City was usually the initial city to really feel the impact. Approximated 2 to 6 Americans died per day during the breakout.

End: It's uncertain what finished the pandemics, yet it might have been the adjustment in climate or quarantines. The last recorded break out in the USA remained in 1911. Immediate cholera treatment is critical, as it can cause fatality. Treatment includes antibiotics, zinc supplements, as well as rehydration.

Now: Cholera still creates virtually 130,000 deaths a year worldwide, according to the CDC. Modern sewage and also water treatment has aided eliminated cholera in some nations, but the virus is still existing somewhere else.
You can get an injection for cholera if you're planning to travel to high-risk locations. The most effective means to avoid cholera is to wash hands routinely with soap as well as water, as well as prevent alcohol consumption contaminated water.

1858: Scarlet fever also can be found in waves

Scarlet fever is a bacterial infection that can happen after strep throat. Like cholera, scarlet fever epidemics were spread in waves. This epidemic disease mainly caught 95 % of children in 1858.

End: Older research studies say that scarlet fever decreased due to enhanced nourishment, but research study shows that improvements in public health were more likely the cause.

Currently: There is no vaccination to prevent strep throat or scarlet fever. It is very important for those with strep throat signs to seek treatment as promptly as feasible. Your medical professional will generally deal with scarlet high temperatures with anti-biotics.

1906-1907: "Typhoid, Mary."

One of the greatest typhoid fever epidemics of perpetuity broke out between 1906 and also 1907 in New York. Mary Mallon, often referred to as "Typhoid Mary," spread out the virus to regarding 122 New Yorkers throughout her time as a cook on an estate as well as in a healthcare facility system. Regarding 5 of those 122, New Yorkers died from the virus. Every year, 10,771 people died from typhoid high temperature.

Clinical screening showed that Mallon was a healthy and balanced provider for typhoid high temperature. Typhoid high temperature creates health issues and red spots to form on the breast and also abdomen.

End: A vaccine was created in 1911, as well as antibiotic therapy for typhoid fever became available in 1948.

Currently: Today, typhoid fever is unusual. Yet it can spread out through direct contact with infected people, as well as the usage of polluted food or water.

1918: "Spanish influenza."

This altering influenza infection, in fact, doesn't originate from Spain. It flows the globe yearly but seriously influenced the United States in 1918. Influenza would return later in 1957 as the "Oriental influenza" and trigger nearly 70,000 deaths prior to an injection appeared.

End: After completion of World war, cases of influenza slowly declined. None of the tips offered at the time, from using masks to drinking coal oil, worked treatments. Today's treatments consist of bed remainder, fluids, as well as antiviral drugs.
Currently: Flu stress mutate each year, making in 2015's inoculations much less effective. It's vital to get your annual vaccination to lower your threat for influenza.

1921-1925: Diphtheria epidemic

Diphtheria peaked in 1921, with 206,000 cases. Diphtheria triggers swelling of the mucous membranes, consisting of in your throat that can obstruct breathing and also ingesting. Often a microbial toxin can go into the bloodstream as well as fatal cause heart and also nerve damage.

End: By the mid-1920s, scientists certified a vaccine against the bacterial illness. Infection rates plunged in the United States.

Now: Today, greater than 80 percent of children in the USA are immunized. Those who contract the disease are treated with anti-biotics.

1916-1955: The height of the polio

Polio is a viral condition that affects the nerves, triggering paralysis. It spreads with direct contact with individuals who have the infection. The first major polio epidemic in the USA occurred in 1916 as well as additionally reached its height in 1952. Of the 57,628 reported cases, there were 3,145 fatalities.

End: Three years later on, Dr. Jonas Salk established a vaccine. By 1962, the ordinary number of cases dropped to 910. The CDC records that the USA has been polio-free given that 1979.

Now: Getting immunized is essential prior to travelling. There's no treatment for polio. Treatment includes enhancing comfort levels and also stopping difficulties.

1981-1991: Measles

Measles is an infection that creates a fever, drippy nose, cough, red eyes, as well as sore throat, as well as later a rash that tops the whole body. It's a really infectious illness as well as can spread out through the air. In the early 20th century, the majority of situations entailed youngsters, due to insufficient vaccination insurance coverage.
End: Doctors started to recommend a second vaccine for every person. Since then, each year has had less than 1,000 situations.

Currently: The USA experienced an additional episode of measles in 2014 as well as 2015. The CDC records that this outbreak was identical to the measles episode in the Philippines in 2014. Make sure to get all the vaccinations your doctor recommends.

1993: Polluted water in Milwaukee

Among Milwaukee's two water treatment plants ended up being contaminated with cryptosporidium, a parasitical condition that causes dehydration, fever, tummy pains, as well as diarrhea. Concerning 403,000 became ill, and more than 100 individuals died, making it the biggest waterborne outbreak in USA background.

End: Lots of people recouped by themselves. Of the people that passed, the majority had actually compromised body immune systems.

Currently: Improved water filtrations aided eliminate this disease. However, approximately 748,000 cases of cryptosporidium still occur annually. Cryptosporidium spreads through dirt, food, water, or contact with contaminated feces. Be sure to practice personal health, particularly when outdoor camping.

2010, 2014: Whooping cough

Pertussis, referred to as whooping coughing, is extremely transmittable as well as among one of the most frequently happening conditions in the USA. These coughing assaults can last for months. Babies also young for inoculation have the greatest danger for life-threatening cases. Ten babies passed away throughout the initial outbreak.
End: A whooping coughing episode comes every three to 5 years. The CDC reports that a rise in the number of situations will likely be the "new normal."

Currently: The occurrence of the illness is a lot less than it was. The CDC suggests that expecting women to get an inoculation throughout the third trimester to enhance defense at birth.

The 1980s to existing: The leading cause of sudden death

First recorded in 1981, the epidemic we now know as HIV first appeared to be an uncommon lung infection. Currently, we know that HIV harms the body's immune system as well as compromises its capability to fight off infections. AIDS is the final stage of HIV and also the 6th leading cause of death in the United States amongst people 25 to 44 years old. HIV might be sent sexually or through blood/body liquids from one person to another. It can be sent from mother to coming baby otherwise treated.

Currently: While there is no remedy for HIV, you can lower your risk via precaution, like making certain your needles are sterilized as well as having safeguarded sex. Precaution can be taken while pregnant to stop the condition from being transferred from an infected mother to a kid. For emergency situations, PEP (post-exposure prophylaxis) is a new antiretroviral medication that stops HIV from creating within 72 hours. Educating yourself regarding existing illness breakouts ought to aid you to comprehend what precautions you to take in order to maintain you and also your household risk-free and also healthy and balanced. Put in the time to search for continuous epidemics by visiting the CDC's Current Episode Checklist, particularly if you are taking a trip.

Protect on your own and your family

Fortunately is that the breakouts detailed here are rare and, in many cases, avoidable. Make certain your family is up to date on their vaccinations before taking a trip, and also obtain the most recent flu inoculation. Easy steps in the kitchen and food safety methods can likewise prevent you and your family members from contracting or transferring infections.

How to respond to an epidemic situation

The list below response suggestions is made use of to arrange concepts, and also to see to it no vital point is forgotten. In this handbook, details ideas are noted for each and every condition, which will help keep the focus on essential elements of each reaction. They are organized into four main blocks:

- Working with responders (C).
- Health and Wellness Information (HEY).
- Communicating threat (C).
- Wellness Interventions (HI).

The checklists will help you analyze what is important and also required for the response. The outbreak feedback varies depending upon the disease. For some diseases, treatment is important; for various other conditions, inoculation is essential.

Coordinating responders

An outbreak is necessarily an exceptional occasion that typically requires extra human and financial resources as well as might also count on added companions, agencies, and also other markets. Solid control is necessary whatsoever times to make sure that all those resources and also partners are working efficiently together to control the breakout. That is commonly expected to lead the worldwide response to sustain national health and wellness authorities. Reliable coordination requires a specialized physical space (usually an emergency operation center); numerous devices to make sure optimum company of conferences as well as filing of documents(such as a checklist of calls, and also a conferences tracking system); a joint strategy frequently upgraded as the situation progresses, to define the treatments required and the distribution of duties as well as obligations amongst stakeholders; and also lastly tools to guarantee interaction in between the various stakeholders participated in the feedback (contact number, a dashboard, maps, and also a directory site).

Coordinating responders list

· What are the attributes of the event that explain it as a situation?
· Those are individuals, groups as well as organizations who should help the response?
· What should they do? (Regards to the recommendation, features).
· Where can responders satisfy? (Emergency situation operation center).

Wellness Information

In every event, information is essential to check it, determine the effect of interventions as well as to guide decision-making throughout the crisis. There are two certain sorts of details:

- Security of the condition, as well as details on the treatments (process and also outcome indications), which shows the coverage as well as the impact of the interventions being done.

- Security supplies details on the number of cases as well as deaths by period and area (individuals, time, as well as area). Info on the interventions enables knowing which ones are done and what is their coverage and effect.

Interacting risk

During the development of any kind of major break out, situations, as well as fatalities, will certainly boost. An epidemic is the rapid spread of contagious conditions to a multitude of individuals in a given population within a short time period. Likewise, there might well be one more sort of epidemic-- the fast spread of details of all kinds, including rumors, gossip as well as unstable info. We define this sensation as an "infodemic."

Infodemics, like epidemics, can be taken care of. Area public health is a fundamental part of outbreak feedback. It encompasses three primary locations: tracking and also determining health threats, outbreaks examination, as well as activities for mitigation and also control. Similarly, effective monitoring of infodemics will be based on surveillance and also recognizing them, analysis of them, as well as control and reduction measures. Danger interaction is an important treatment in any type of response to condition breakouts and is equally needed to take care of infodemics.

Connecting threat in epidemics entails two-way

Communication that is vibrant and also developing as the outbreak develops. Break out risk communication entails three main strands that must work together.

1. Talk. Authorities, experts, and also reaction groups, should quickly pass on information on the nature of the event as well as the protective steps that people can take.

2. We can use social mobilizers and frontline responders; motivate area engagement; along with in-person interaction using relied on interlocutors such as community leaders, spiritual numbers as well as area wellness workers. We should utilize translational interaction techniques to develop messages that are appropriate for the target populations in regards to language, educational degree as well as social contexts.

3. Listen. Responders, professionals as well as authorities must promptly examine and also understand the worries, problems, assumptions and also sights of those affected; and also customize their interventions and messages to attend to such worries. This calls for making use of social science research as well as neighborhood interaction expertise as well as methods.

4. Manage rumors. Disease breakouts are commonly accompanied by the visibility of false rumors as well as false information. -responders need to have ways to listen to such false information as well as

appropriate instances of it in ideal means immediately.

Wellness Interventions

Each illness calls for a various collection of wellness treatments to decrease transmission, serious morbidity as well as death the effect on health and wellness systems as well as also on the political and various other industries.

The Emergency Situation Response Structure (ERF) is an interior WHO tool that lays out a collection of treatments to better reply to emergencies. Under this structure, for any kind of emergency that requires WHO operational feedback, the Organization turns on the Event Monitoring System (IMS), recognized the finest practice for emergency situation monitoring. WHO has adjusted the IMS to consist of 6 vital functions? The four blocks and feedback ideas are integrated right into the Incident Management System. Although all six features of the IMS are critical for successful action, the four blocks will certainly highlight what specifies for each and every condition.

ABOUT THE AUTHOR

Matthew Coleridge was born in Texas and he took place in many volunteer actions for emergency situations in natural disasters. With his volunteering actions he saved a lot of people's lives and faced different dangerous survival situations. During these scenarios, he has always known how to maintain calm and adapt to every situation. After his retirement, he decided to share his survival skills and knowledge in first aid and nursing.

www.ingramcontent.com/pod-product-compliance
Lightning Source LLC
Chambersburg PA
CBHW050010230526
45465CB00003BB/1345